ANIMAL
INVESTIGATORS

How the World's First Wildlife Forensics Lab
Is Solving Crimes and Saving Endangered Species

Laurel A. Neme, Ph.D.

FOREWORD BY
Richard Leakey

SCRIBNER
New York London Toronto Sydney

SCRIBNER
A Division of Simon & Schuster, Inc.
1230 Avenue of the Americas
New York, NY 10020

Manufactured in the United States of America

ISBN-13: 978-1-4165-5056-3

To Mom Pom and Dad Pad
Who taught me by example to follow my dreams

CONTENTS

FOREWORD

As a child growing up in the African bush at Olduvai Gorge, where animal sounds and storybook sights filled my soul, I gained an appreciation of our intimate relationship with and interconnectedness to nature. That realization inspired me to dedicate my life to ensuring that wild animals and places will be around for generations to come.

Since the 1980s, when I worked to stop the elephant slaughter in Kenya and establish a ban on trade in elephant ivory, it has become apparent that illegal wildlife trafficking is threatening the very existence of already endangered plants and animals around the globe. Such trafficking is so massive it ranks a close third in illicit international commerce, behind only drugs and weapons. Ultimately, it cannot be stemmed without both greater investment in enforcement and increased awareness.

Animal Investigators provides an excellent account of how a little-known group of dedicated scientists is providing a new and vital weapon in the arsenal of wildlife law enforcement officers. It is my hope that the telling of their fascinating stories will help generate the public support necessary to expand both their efforts and the work of their colleagues and allies around the world.

RICHARD LEAKEY, renowned paleontologist,
conservationist, and founder of WildlifeDirect

INTRODUCTION

Until the early 1980s, wildlife poachers and smugglers had an easy time getting away with murder. U.S. Fish and Wildlife Service (FWS) special agent Terry Grosz aimed to change that. Since 1976 he'd been the FWS Law Enforcement's endangered species desk officer in charge of facilitating the agency's endangered species investigations nationwide. His agents were tasked with protecting animals such as elephants and rhinoceroses, whose populations were endangered from hunters and middlemen seeking to supply ivory, horn, and other products to consumers worldwide, and he'd quickly grown fed up with seeing suspects avoid prosecution for lack of proof. It wasn't that the agents didn't have the evidence. They just couldn't find anyone who would testify. Scientists who were willing to examine the evidence, such as an ornithologist at a museum or biologist at a research institute or university, typically refused to present and defend their results in court, which was a necessary step for conviction. That made their evaluations worthless.

Even if they had been willing to testify, other complicating matters would have come into play. Unlike regular crime labs, the museums and universities that did the analysis typically had inadequate security and procedures. That meant they could not maintain a secure chain of custody, so that during subsequent legal proceedings the defendant could have argued that the evidence was corrupted. Other times researchers had competing commitments that took precedence, so much so that their results would have arrived too late for trial, or else they could not prove the species of origin, making the results inconclusive and therefore of no use.

Human forensic labs *were* accustomed to testifying in criminal proceedings. Yet no crime lab could justify working an animal case over a human one. After being laughed out of the Federal Bureau of Investigation's (FBI) lab once too often because of its higher-priority human cases, Grosz appealed to anyone who would listen—and even others who wouldn't—for a wildlife crime lab. He lobbied his superiors within FWS and pleaded with others who had influence over the agency, such as Amos Eno, then executive director of the National Fish and Wildlife Foundation (a nonprofit organization established by Congress in 1984 to sustain the nation's fish, wildlife, plants, and habitats through leadership conservation investments) and members of Congress who controlled its budget: FWS needed its own forensic lab dedicated to wildlife.

Forensics applies science to crimes. It is based on the theory that, for virtually every infraction of the law, the suspect, victim, and crime scene interact in such a way as to exchange trace evidence, which can then be analyzed to link the perpetrator to his or her misdeed. By establishing a wildlife crime lab, Grosz hoped to put a damper on the rampant illegal killing of wild animals.

Killing wild animals is big business. While much wildlife trade is legal, a huge black market exists, especially in rare and endangered species. Legal trade in animals, which ranges from reptilian leather goods to pets like tropical fish and turtles to seafood and meat, amounts to about $15 billion to $55 billion a year. Of this, the United States processes about $2.8 billion in shipments a year. However, that figure reflects only wildlife consignments that are reported by the importer to authorities. An unknown volume of wildlife cargo is never declared, meaning that a booming illegal trade takes place outside official channels.

Illegal wildlife trafficking is worth perhaps $20 billion annually, and some say more. It is the third most lucrative criminal trade in the world, ranking behind drugs and human trafficking and in front of arms smuggling. Ounce for ounce, illicit products such as rhino horn and deer musk can be worth more than gold, diamonds, or cocaine and other drugs. In the 1990s, crystallized bear bile sold in South Korea for over $1,000 a gram, about twenty times the price of heroin.

The number and diversity of illegal wildlife products is huge, including everything from exotic pets, such as live primates, birds, and reptiles, to traditional Chinese medicines, art, and high-fashion accessories made from animal parts. The United States is both one of the world's largest markets for illegal wildlife and wildlife products, with many believing it ranks second only to China, as well as one of the largest suppliers. Yet the scope of the problem is really global, with both illicit and legal products and animal parts passing from east to west, developing to developed countries, and vice versa. For example, endangered Tibetan antelopes, known as chiru, are killed for their wool, which is then woven into soft, thin shahtoosh shawls destined for New York and Europe's fashion elite. A single shawl, worth up to $15,000, uses the wool from five slaughtered animals. In Caspian Sea countries like Russia, sturgeon eggs are cut from these protected prehistoric fish as a culinary delicacy. The caviar, some of which is legal and some illegal, is then sold in Europe and New York for over $2,000 for a small 250-gram tin. South America's rare reptiles are processed into boots, purses, and belts, while endangered primates from Africa both feed the growing domestic market for bushmeat and supply the foreign market for exotic pets. And literally tons of legal and illegal wildlife products are used for traditional medicine in China and the rest of Asia.

Thousands of species and millions of animals are affected by wildlife trade. Over 25,000 primates, 2 to 3 million birds, 10 million reptile skins, and over 500 million tropical fish are legally traded each year.[1] Law enforcement and other experts suggest illegal wildlife trade may equal the legal trade, although comprehensive statistics detailing the magnitude of wildlife crime are unavailable. Agencies such as Interpol, the World Customs Organization, the European Union, and the Convention on International Trade in Endangered Species of Wild Fauna and Flora (CITES) maintain databases, but they are incomplete because reporting is inconsistent and much illicit trade goes undetected.

When the International Fund for Animal Welfare (IFAW) in 2008 tracked more than 7,000 online auctions and advertisements in eight countries that offered protected wildlife and wildlife products for sale, it estimated 91 percent of the trade was probably illegal.[2] The products included rugs, from leopard, tiger, and polar bear skins, tiger teeth and claws; live exotic birds such as double yellow-headed and yellow-naped Amazon parrots, scarlet macaws and hyacinth macaws; live tortoises and big snakes; sea turtle products, crocodile-leather items such as purses and briefcases; a $23,000 bowl made from rhinoceros horn; and more than 5,000 elephant ivory products ranging from calling card cases to figurines. The scope and variety of the illegal trade is immense, and nearly all protected species, especially exotic ones, are affected.

The reason for the illegal trade's prevalence is simple: a trifecta of low risk, weak penalties, and high profits. By and large, poachers and traders have little fear of getting caught. The vast size of most wilderness areas and the limited number of enforcement officers virtually guarantee them free access. Even when violators are arrested and convicted, they suffer few consequences, from confiscation of the property or denial of gun ownership or hunting rights to small fines or, on occasion, imprisonment. By comparison, profits can be astronomical. Earnings from illegal wildlife trafficking often amount to well over a 1,000 percent return on investment.

Illicit profits swell exponentially the farther the animal travels both from its origin and original form. For a single rhinoceros horn, a destitute hunter in Africa could earn several hundred dollars, the equivalent of a year's salary,[3] but "processing" the product boosts its value. The same rhinoceros horn, ground up and included in remedies for male impotence or other ailments, could fetch half a million dollars in the Asian market.[4]

The high payoffs and low risks from wildlife trafficking attract a wide variety of criminals, from petty lawbreakers to sophisticated international terrorists. Increasingly, law enforcement officers see wildlife trafficking cases that exhibit a high degree of detailed planning (for recruiting, equipping, and paying poachers), sophisticated smuggling techniques (such as forging documents and ingenious cargo concealment), and cross-border movement, which suggest that organized crime groups are becoming more involved in the business. As evidence of this connection, William Clark, chairman of the Interpol Working Group on Wildlife Crime since 1994, points to a "conspicuous increase" in the frequency of seizures of large consignments for a wide variety of contraband—including coral, snake skins, conch shells, shahtoosh, and ivory—that are often characterized as "the largest of this type in history."[5] The seizure of 6.5 tons of elephant ivory in Singapore in 2002 and 3.9 tons seized in Hong Kong in 2006 are two such examples.

These massive illegal shipments are undertakings that require substantial up-front investments to finance the poaching of the animals and the processing and marketing of the illegal goods, and significant organizational capacity to conceal and move the products thousands of miles across multiple borders. The recent ivory seizures exhibit all these characteristics, as DNA analysis indicates that the ivory confiscated in Singapore came from Zambian elephants, even though it had been shipped from Malawi, and the ivory seized in Hong Kong originated from animals in Gabon, even though it had been sent from Cameroon. These features and the complexity of the transactions suggest that organized crime, and not small-time crooks, was behind these gigantic shipments.

Anecdotal evidence also links wildlife trafficking and terrorism, with proceeds from illegal animal trade financing rebel groups. A March 2008 *Newsweek* article described how Sudan's Janjaweed militia, which has been implicated in the Darfur genocide, sold or bartered tusks from hundreds of elephants it poached around Chad's Zakouma National Park to support its activities, and also how a Somali warlord acted similarly by equipping and funding gangs to poach elephants along Kenya's Tana River.[6] In the Democratic Republic of Congo (DRC), illegal trade in ivory and bushmeat provides economic support for rogue military gangs, with the Tshuapa-Lomami-Lualaba Project documenting roughly 14 tons of illegal ivory smuggled from the Okapi Wildlife Reserve area (a UNESCO World Heritage Site) of which two major shipments were chartered by Congolese rebels.[7] And the links between terrorism and illegal wildlife trafficking are not limited to Africa. A May 2007 article in *The Guardian* newspaper (United Kingdom) detailed how al-Qaeda-affiliated Islamic militants are sponsoring poaching in and around Kaziranga National Park, a UNESCO World Heritage Site in northeastern India that is home to over 500 birds and 52 large mammals, including Chinese pangolin, elephants, and rhinoceroses.[8]

These and other reports have prompted significant congressional concern, so much so that on March 5, 2008, the U.S. House of Representatives' Committee on Natural Resources held a hearing on illegal wildlife trafficking, titled "Poaching American Security: Impacts of Illegal Wildlife Trade." At this hearing, House Natural Resources chairman Nick Rahall (D-W. Va.) said the illegal trade was "the wildlife version of blood diamonds."[9]

Spurring the illegal wildlife trade is the fact that endangered animals are often worth more dead than alive. Virtually every part of a tiger, for example, has value. Its bones, which can sell for $400 per kilogram ($175 per pound), are used in traditional Chinese medicine to treat ulcers, typhoid, malaria, dysentery, burns, and even rheumatism. Other parts, like its whiskers, can be worn as talismans or protective charms. Consumers believe its penis gives strength, with one Japanese brand of tiger penis pills selling for $27,000 per bottle in the late 1990s. Its kneecaps are said to cure arthritis, its tail is used to treat skin diseases, and its skin is sold as a trophy or carpet, or worn as clothing to act as a symbol of wealth.[10] Processed and sold separately, parts from a single tiger can be worth as much as $60,000.[11]

Other protected species also fetch high prices. In 2008, the Congressional Research Service reported retail values of up to $900 per kilogram ($408 per pound) for elephant ivory, up to $50,000 per kilogram ($22,680 per pound) for rhino horn, up to $80,000 for a mature breeding pair of black palm cockatoos, and $8,500 for a pair of bird-wing butterflies.[12]

Dwindling populations don't always stop demand. To the contrary, the increasing rarity of a species can simply raise prices and profits . . . and *intensify* its desirability. While traditional craftspeople, for example, treasured elephant ivory and tortoiseshell for their exceptional malleability and luminescence, the availability of plastic and other substitutes did not end demand for these products. Far from it. According to Tom Milliken, Africa program director for TRAFFIC International, during 2006 authorities intercepted over 1,100 illegal ivory shipments, an average of 92 shipments every month.[13] State Department assistant secretary Claudia McMurray confirmed the persistent desirability for ivory when she testified that, despite rising ivory prices (from $200 per kilogram [$91 per pound] in 2005 to up to $900 per kilogram [$408 per pound] in 2008), during a two-week period in January 2008 Namibian authorities seized 200 kilograms (441 pounds) of raw ivory (representing seven dead elephants), Kenyan officials confiscated 80 kilograms (176 pounds) of raw and worked ivory smuggled at the airport, and Zimbabwe police arrested eleven poachers suspected of killing 15 elephants in Hwange National Park.[14] These incidents show demand for ivory remains strong, and demonstrate that the animal's scarcity may have merely heightened its cachet.

The result is overexploitation at a time when factors such as habitat loss and global warming threaten those same species. While estimates vary, experts believe extinctions are happening between 50 and 1,000 times faster than what is considered the natural rate. According to the

Red List of Threatened Species, compiled by the International Union for Conservation of Nature (IUCN), over 16,000 plant and animal species, including one in four mammals, one in eight birds, and one in three amphibians, face a high risk of extinction soon, largely from human activities. It is the greatest mass extinction, and the first human-induced one, since the age of the dinosaurs.

Illegal wildlife trade hastens these trends.

The illicit trade in ivory demonstrates the stark effect it can have on a species. From 1979 to 1989, illegal poaching to augment the legally allowed trade of ivory decimated African elephant populations, reducing their numbers from 1.2 million to 600,000—a 50 percent drop in just ten years. Tigers, rhinoceros, Tibetan antelope, and Asian black bears, among others, have seen similar dramatic declines, largely from illegal trade in their parts. As State Department assistant secretary McMurray warned at the March 2008 congressional hearing, "Illegal wildlife trade has brought us to a 'tipping point'" that is driving many species to the brink of extinction.[15]

When only small numbers of endangered species remain, killing even a single animal drastically reduces the species' chances for survival. In Cambodia, for instance, the deputy head of the Forestry Protection department, Sun Hean, lamented that the 200 tigers poached over a five-year period in the early 2000s cut the country's entire tiger population in half.[16] With only a couple hundred animals remaining, the possibility of breeding and increasing the population is poor, and it may not be long before Cambodia has no tigers at all.

The overexploitation of wildlife for commerce has a long history that, ultimately, prompted legal restrictions on the trade. At the turn of the nineteenth century, nations watched their fish and wildlife populations drop sharply in order to supply demand from both inside and outside their countries. From 1870 to 1920, tens of millions of birds died around the world to adorn high-fashion hats and clothing, with over one million skins of either herons or egrets, the species most severely damaged, sold between 1897 and 1911, according to a single London auction record.[17] Similarly, in India, hunters killed at least 80,000 tigers between 1875 and 1925 to earn the bounty offered by British colonizers, who viewed the animals as pests.[18]

Internationally, the legal reaction began with two unsuccessful attempts by colonial powers to preserve big-game hunting grounds: the 1900 London Convention Designed to Ensure the Conservation of Various Species of Wild Animals in Africa Which Are Useful to Man or Inoffensive; and the 1933 London Convention Relative to the Preservation of Fauna and Flora in Their Natural State. Both treaties harmonized local wildlife management rules and addressed the problem of unsustainable wildlife exploitation through a basic system of hunting restrictions and controls for threatened species. However, neither came to fruition. The first (the 1900 Convention) was not ratified by all the signatories, so it never entered into force, and the second failed due to the lack of institutions for decision-making and day-to-day operations as well as impending decolonization. The problem of gaining full support from all parties and adequate enforcement has proven to be a persistent one. Two regional treaties, the 1940 Washington Convention on Nature Protection and Wild Life Preservation in the Western Hemisphere and the 1968 Algiers African Convention on the Conservation of Nature and Natural Resources, followed, but the responsible organizations (the Organization of American States and the Organization of African Unity, respectively) never effectively implemented them.[19]

In the United States, similar concern about animal overexploitation led to passage of the nation's first wildlife protection law, the Lacey Act of 1900, which prohibited interstate commerce in illegally taken wildlife and banned the importation of harmful species. It was soon followed by the 1918 Migratory Bird Treaty Act, which regulated migratory bird hunting and made it illegal to take, possess, buy, sell, purchase, or barter in migratory birds, feathers, parts, nests, or eggs of these birds. In 1930, the Tariff Act required a certificate of legal acquisition for imports of bird and mammals and their parts, and in 1935, the Lacey Act was extended to include wildlife imported from abroad.

Yet the massive slaughter of animals for international trade continued unabated. From the early 1950s to 1960s, hunters and traders decimated previously abundant reptile populations in South America for their hides, exporting them to Europe and the United States for shoes, handbags, and luggage. In 1950, hunters took 12 million black caiman (*Melanosuchus niger*) skins from the Amazon Basin alone. While the reptile trade generally targeted South American species, it also included crocodiles from Africa, Asia, and Australia, and led to the near extinction of the American alligator (*Alligator mississippiensis*). In fact, during the 1950s and early 1960s the trade in reptile products depleted about 85 percent of the world's crocodilians.[20] In response, many U.S. states banned the killing of American alligators and trade in their hides, and Brazil and other South American countries prohibited caiman exports.

While these efforts were helpful, governments and environmental groups realized that controlling exports could not work without equal attention to the demand side of the equation. The first formal cry for a comprehensive wildlife trade system came in 1963 at the General Assembly of the IUCN, the world's first global environmental organization that now comprises over 1,000 governments and nongovernmental organizations and 10,000 volunteer scientists in more than 160 countries. At that meeting, members called for an "international convention on regulation of export, transit and import of rare or threatened wildlife species or their skins and trophies."

Meanwhile, the United States continued to refine its wildlife legislation and, in 1969, passed the Endangered Species Conservation Act, which ordered the development of a list of wildlife threatened with worldwide extinction and bans to their commercial import. Yet the American fur and leather industries and those involved in the pet trade feared this act would put them at a competitive disadvantage globally. Congress addressed these fears by directing the U.S. government to work toward enacting similar laws in other countries, and said it should convene a high-level international meeting with the aim of negotiating a binding international treaty for the conservation of endangered species.

The IUCN had prepared and circulated several treaty drafts to governments and nongovernmental organizations since its 1963 General Assembly, with each controlling wildlife trade through global lists of threatened species drawn up and updated by a committee of international experts. However, several countries, namely big wildlife exporters in the developing world, led by Kenya, and the United States opposed this approach, arguing instead that each country should develop its own lists.

The two approaches were consolidated in a 1972 treaty draft, which then served as the working document for an international Conference of Plenipotentiaries held at the Pentagon in Washington, D.C., from February 12 to March 3, 1973. The resulting legally binding treaty, signed by eighty countries, was the Convention on International Trade in Endangered Species of Wild Fauna and Flora, which entered into force in 1975 after its tenth ratification.

Often called a "Magna Carta for wildlife," CITES regulates international trade in listed species in order to prevent or address their over-exploitation and illegal trade. It prohibits commercial trade in the most imperiled plants and animals and controls trade of those still at risk but less so. Legal CITES trade is based on two preconditions: a legal acquisition finding, and a finding that the trade will not be detrimental to the survival of the species in the wild.

Currently, CITES protects about 5,000 animal species (with bans for around 600) and 28,000 plant species. Trade restrictions are based on scientific assessments of the threat to a species' sustainability from international commerce. These assessments are then used as the basis for deciding to list a species in its three Appendices to the Convention, each of which provides different levels of trade protection based on the species' conservation status.

CITES recognizes that trade prohibitions and regulations can succeed only if the export restrictions of supplying nations are supported by the import restrictions of buying ones. This twofold approach, with enforceable controls at both the exit point (country of origin) and final destination, applies to over 170 signatory nations to make CITES arguably the most successful multilateral environmental agreement.

In general, enforcement is carried out by the signatories' own national laws and agencies. In the United States, Congress passed the Endangered Species Act (ESA) in 1973, in large part to enforce CITES. The ESA expanded the scope of previous wildlife protection laws (and replaced the Endangered Species Conservation Act of 1969) to regulate not only the import but also the export, taking, possession, and commercial trade of both endangered and threatened foreign and domestic species.

The bulk of responsibility for implementation of the Endangered Species Act went to the Fish and Wildlife Service in the U.S. Department of Interior. For the thirty years prior to the 1973 enactment of the ESA, however, FWS had primarily managed game and enforced hunting regulations. To enforce this broader and more complex mandate, FWS extended the role of its officers from the equivalent of uniformed patrol officers, or "duck cops" as they were known, looking for violations, to plainclothes detectives redefined as "special agents," who would investigate wildlife crimes after the fact.

Special agents' focus on wildlife trafficking expanded the types of relevant evidence collected to increasingly include animal parts and processed products. But agents had a big problem. To prove commission of a crime, they had to establish that the sales were illegal, and to do that, they had to show the evidence came from a *protected* species, which was easier said than done.

After several years of political wrangling, in 1979 Grosz's persistence paid off when FWS agreed to hire a lab director who would set up a forensics program for wildlife law enforcement. After over half a dozen candidates were interviewed, the last one, Ken Goddard, a crime lab director, biochemist, and chief criminologist from Southern California's Huntington Beach Police Department, met with FWS Law Enforcement chief Clark Bavin and Special Agent Grosz. At the interview, Bavin and Grosz grilled Goddard to test his way of thinking. For the final question, as he had with all the others, Grosz complained about political opposition to the lab and asked whether Goddard would fudge the scientific evaluation in order to ensure that the lab "won" several times in a row and thus quell agents' hostility by proving the lab's utility. Furious, Goddard threatened to report anyone who asked him to falsify results and walked out of the interview.

Goddard assumed he wouldn't get the job. But he was wrong. The lab's credibility depended on its being above reproach and never taking evidence further than it went. Six months later, FWS offered Goddard the job.

For the next ten years, Goddard worked out of his briefcase, following the agents, analyzing evidence, and advocating for the creation of the lab. In 1985, Congress allocated $1 million to establish an actual lab. Finally, in 1989, with an additional $3.5 million for construction and purchasing of equipment, the U.S. Fish and Wildlife Service Forensics Laboratory, dubbed the "Scotland Yard of wildlife crime," officially opened its doors in Ashland, Oregon.

Since then, it's grown from just ten forensic scientists to a staff of more than thirty-five. The lab's caseload has also grown, from about 80 cases in its first year to an average of 600 cases annually now, with each case typically involving numerous, often hundreds, of separate pieces of evidence that need to be analyzed. During the first eighteen years of operation, the lab worked on over 9,500 cases and analyzed roughly 68,000 pieces of evidence.[21]

As with any crime lab, the wildlife forensics lab and its scientists have two jobs: first, to identify evidence; and second, to link the suspect and crime scene. Like standard police labs, it uses physical evidence such as fingerprints, tire tracks, bullets, gunshot residue, poisons, and DNA to reveal what might have happened to its animal victims and to identify possible suspects. But this lab has an extra job: figuring out *what* the victim is.

The lab handles over 30,000 species of victims, which makes a regular police lab, with a mere *one* species to worry about, look like a vacation spot. The lab's staff aren't just working feverishly to solve crimes, they are forging a new field of science as they go. Not only does the lab handle a vast array of species, it also has to work from a vast array of products and specimens—victims often arrive as unidentifiable parts, a carved statuette or a belt or a small vial of pills—that give no clue to the victims' identity. As lab director Goddard explains, "All the things that might tell you 'this is an elephant' aren't there."[22] The scientific challenge is often to reverse the manufacturing process, to trace a product back to the species from which it came.

Identification of species is vital for enforcing the law. Because legal protections for animals are based on the species, agents must substantiate their accusations against a suspect by proving beyond a reasonable doubt that the animal involved is in fact a species that is listed. For live animals, that's not difficult because acceptable species-defining characteristics are already well established by scientists. But for wildlife parts and processed products found in commercial trade, that's not the case. Without a definition of species contained in parts and derivative products that is accepted by the scientific community and in court, agents can't prove crimes exist, suspects go free, and their illegal contraband is freely traded on the market.

The lab's job is to create scientifically defensible and legally acceptable definitions of species for wildlife parts and products. As Goddard notes, "If you can't legally define what a species is, you can't protect it."[23] Hence, the lab must figure out what techniques to apply to the evidence, identify a unique characteristic contained in the animal part in question, and then develop a methodology that finds that trait consistently. All of this takes time, often years, and requires a highly specific knowledge of the species.

A single piece of evidence might be handled by several of the lab's seven teams. The *morphology* unit examines items like fur, hides, feathers, claws, and teeth both visually and microscopically and then uses their form and structure to determine what species they came from. *Criminalistics* analyzes trace evidence found at crime scenes, such as fingerprints, bullets, and tool marks, to find out what happened to the victim. Using equipment like electron microscopes, mass spectrometers, and liquid chromatographs, the *chemistry* team assesses the elemental components of animal blood and tissue from a range of products, like organs and powdered medicines, while *genetics* analyzes DNA to identify both species and individuals. When the victim is relatively intact, *pathology* performs a necropsy (animal autopsy) on the carcass to ascertain the cause and process of death. In addition, the lab's *digital evidence* unit analyzes computer, audio, and video evidence and helps develop court displays. Finally, the evidence control unit of the *administrative* branch supports the lab staff by controlling evidence handling (i.e., ensuring a secure and unbroken chain of custody) and other tasks.

Today, with Goddard at the helm, the wildlife forensics laboratory works as part of FWS to achieve the agency's overall objective of conserving, protecting, and enhancing the nation's fish and wildlife and their habitats, for the continuing benefit of the American people. Specifically, it helps identify the species or subspecies of pieces, parts, and products of an animal; determine the cause of death of an animal; assist wildlife officers in determining if a violation of the law occurred; and identify and compare physical evidence to try to link suspect, victim, and crime scene. The lab's work is vital to FWS's mission of enforcing federal wildlife laws and protecting endangered species.

Before the wildlife crime lab, when the legally protected animal left the poacher's hands, the prospects for prosecution grew slimmer and slimmer as the victim was plucked, boiled, sliced, and diced until transformed into its end product. Now when it's time to go to court, the lab adds credibility to the evidence so that agents get convictions. As Grosz puts it, "It's a hell of a hammer."[24] The lab's DNA analysis of sturgeon eggs led to the January 2001 conviction and imprisonment of a New York City–based food importer for selling phony Russian caviar.[25] Similarly, the lab's identification of hair from Tibetan antelopes led to the 2000 guilty plea of Hong Kong– and U.S.-based shahtoosh dealers in a judicial proceeding where dozens of shawl owners, including supermodel Christie Brinkley, were subpoenaed to testify about the illegal sales. Each year, agents' cases result in the prosecution of around 10,000 civil and criminal violations, and the lab's analysis helps to prove these crimes and, consequently, reduce illegal wildlife trade.

The lab works with roughly 200 federal wildlife law enforcement agents, all fifty state fish and game agencies, and the more than 170 foreign countries that signed CITES. Its modern, newly expanded 40,000-square-foot building, situated on the campus of Southern Oregon University (formerly known as Southern Oregon State College) in Ashland boasts a state-of-the-art lab unlike any other. The liquid nitrogen freezer sits unobtrusively up against the far wall, but crack it open and, after the clouds clear, you'll see stacks of animal blood and tissue samples that are used to differentiate wildlife species down to the cellular level. Enter the walk-in freezer off the evidence room, which features feathers, hides, bones, and preserved animals, and you'll find animal parts and full carcasses awaiting examination. In the lab's new "bug" room, peer into a coffin-sized Plexiglas box holding thousands of black carpet (dermestid) beetles as they busily swarm over bones, cleaning them without altering evidence of trauma such as tool marks.

In the conference room, a wall of open bookcases, what Goddard calls the "shop of horrors," offers a seemingly endless collection of the fruits of wildlife poaching: polar bear rugs, tarantula paperweights, sea turtle–shell lamps, a crocodile-face ashtray, and cobra-skin cowboy boots with shriveled heads rising from each tip like hood ornaments. And in the "men's corner," the shelves of dried seal penises, bear paws, and various potions and pills allegedly made from rhino horn, tiger bone, or musk—all whipped up to counteract male impotence—make one wonder if Viagra might inadvertently be the savior of wildlife.

This book brings the reader inside the lab's day-to-day operation to show how its groundbreaking identification work protects species. We'll watch as the scientists pursue three cases. First, the case of Alaskan walrus slaughtered for their ivory, which is made more complex by the role of the Native Eskimo people whose culture and livelihood are centered on the hunt. Next, an investigation of the trade in black bear gallbladders used in traditional Chinese medicine; a brutal case involving animal cruelty in the service of greed. Finally, we'll explore the world of illegal smuggling of Brazilian Amazon feather art that exploits the Indians who make it and threatens jaguars, scarlet macaws, harpy eagles, and other protected tropical animals.

We'll see how the scientists at the world's first and only full-service crime laboratory dedicated to wildlife develop new protocols as they go. With each case and each analysis, they not only expand the infant field of wildlife forensics but also lessen the chance that poachers and smugglers will get away with murder.

CHAPTER ONE

Native Alaskan
Subsistence Hunting

The big lump didn't move. From a distance, it looked like a brown boulder, but Tim Asigrook* knew this flat stretch of beach contained nothing larger than the pebbles in his rock collection. He revved the engine of his four-wheeler and sped closer, stopping upwind where the smell wasn't quite as nauseating. As he climbed off the vehicle and made his way to the huge mass, his eyes confirmed what his heart already knew: it was a dead, headless walrus.

For most of the six hundred people in his Siberian Yup'ik village of Gambell, Alaska, a wasted walrus like this one was an affront. For over two thousand years, Asigrook's people had survived on wind-shattered St. Lawrence Island—located in the Bering Sea two hundred miles from Nome, the closest city on the Alaska mainland, and thirty-eight miles from the Chukchi Peninsula in Russia—by hunting marine mammals such as walrus, whale, and seal for their basic necessities: food, clothing, and shelter.

Fifty-year-old Asigrook, like most Native Alaskan hunters, typically brought back as much of an animal as he could transport. Even as modern conveniences reached the remote island and the villagers' needs changed, they still used as much of the animal as possible—meat, hide, and ivory. Not to do so would be wasteful and would defy thousands of years of tradition.

Hunting was more than an economic necessity for Alaskan Natives like Asigrook; it was a spiritual tradition that fed their souls as well as their bodies. The way they hunted defined them. Their relationship

*Not his actual name.

1

with, and treatment of, the animals shaped their identities, from their language, art, clothing, legends, and celebrations, to their beliefs about community, economy, and spirituality.

Native hunters perceived their animal quarries as equals and their success depended on showing respect for the soul of their prey. They believed the mammals gifted themselves willingly to the hunters of their choosing and that this self-sacrifice represented an act of sharing and rebirth.[1] This reverence for nature and belief in transformation was not unique. Many traditional cultures, such as Native Americans in the southwest United States and indigenous Indians in Brazil, shared similar views. To the Alaskan Natives, when a hunter killed a walrus, he did not conquer it. Rather, he created a bond between his people and the environment. If he failed to respect this relationship, he'd offend the animals, who would then disappear and, in turn, threaten the future survival of the hunter and his family. The hunt was a mutual tribute between man and mammal.

Asigrook shook his head at the carnage. The bloated carcass lay just at the water's edge where it had been cast by wind and waves. The large animal was basically intact, except for where its distinctive head

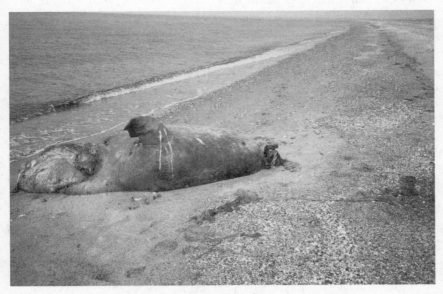

Headless walrus washed up on beach. *(Courtesy of Laurel A. Neme)*

and tusks used to be. There, instead of a bulbous face and whiskers, shiny white bone poked from the mass of rotting muscle.

The dangerous weather may have forced hunters to leave quickly and take only the easiest and most valuable part of the animal. Or it could have been that this walrus had been lost during the initial kill and found later when virtually everything but the tusks was rotten, making the head the only part of the animal worth salvaging.

Yet Asigrook feared the worst: that it had been deliberately killed solely for the ivory.

Killing, selling, and importing marine mammals and their parts and products is forbidden under the 1972 Marine Mammal Protection Act (MMPA). This law came about in response to concerns among scientists that human activities were depleting marine mammal species as well as the public's outcry about the hunting of seal pups in the North Atlantic and the high incidental catches of dolphins by tuna fisheries. Unintentional catches from commercial fishing substantially reduced dolphin populations, and over 100,000 died each year during the 1970s and early 1980s when trapped in tuna nets. Populations of northern fur seals, harbor seals, and Steller sea lions also suffered from their accidental catch in fishing operations, while other marine mammals such as the southern sea otter were hunted almost to extinction for their fur. The Marine Mammal Protection Act was the first law to mandate an ecosystem approach to marine resource management. As such, it protected an entire category of wildlife regardless of its population status. While walrus are not threatened or endangered, they are legally protected under this law. They are also listed under CITES Appendix III (at the request of Canada), which regulates international trade of walrus products by requiring appropriate permits or certificates.

Responsibility for enforcing the Marine Mammal Protection Act is divided between FWS, which oversees sea otters, manatees, dugong (which are similar in behavior and appearance to manatees), walrus, and polar bears, and the National Marine Fisheries Service (NMFS) in the Department of Commerce, which oversees cetaceans (whales, porpoises, and dolphins) and all pinnipeds (seals and sea lions) except for walrus.

Under the act, limited numbers of marine mammals can be collected for scientific and public display purposes, and some caught unintentionally by commercial fishing operations are allowed. An exemption gives Alaskan Natives the right to hunt walrus *provided they do so for subsistence and not in a way that is "wasteful."* While "wasteful" is a relative term and still a subject of contention, both Native Alaskans and federal law enforcement largely agree that killing a walrus just for its tusks, or headhunting, is wasteful and therefore illegal.

Walrus tusks are modified canine teeth that range in size and weight. While they can grow to over three feet long in males (two feet in females), the length of most tusks averages about 16 inches. The shape of male and female tusks differs slightly. Bull tusks tend to be straighter, thicker (1¼ to 2½ inches wide at the base), and heavier (between two to three pounds each) than those of females. While of similar length, female tusks are more slender (1½ inches at the base) and consequently weigh less (about one to two pounds). A cross section would also reveal a more rounded shape for female tusks and a more oval one for males.

The classic ivory appearance comes from the tusk's outer primary dentin layer. Underneath is a secondary dentin layer that possesses a "marbled" or oatmeal-like appearance unique to walrus and valued by Native Alaskans for their intricate carvings.

Asigrook couldn't accept hunters killing walrus only for their ivory, but he understood it. Traditionally, his people had eaten the walrus meat and fed some to their sled dogs; used the hides for skin-covered boats, shelter, and clothes; refined the blubber into cooking and fuel oil (prior to the 1940s); constructed houses with the bones; and carved the ivory tusks into tools such as harpoon points for hunting, or works of art they could sell. But times had changed. Their island was less iso-

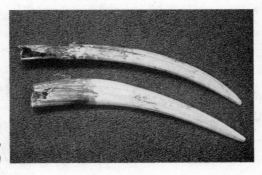

Raw walrus tusks.
(Courtesy of U.S. Fish and Wildlife Service Forensics Laboratory)

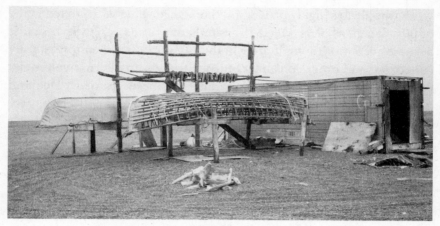

Examples of traditional walrus-skin boats, Gambell, Alaska. *(Courtesy of Laurel A. Neme)*

lated than it used to be. They got electricity and telephone service in the 1970s, and over the years gained greater access to running water and a variety of foods and other consumer goods. Now they used plastic buckets rather than painstakingly crafting containers from walrus stomachs. They bought waterproof raincoats instead of spending weeks making them from walrus intestines. They built their houses with wood, cement, and tin instead of using walrus and whale bones and skin. They used aluminum motorboats in addition to their traditional walrus-skin boats for hunting and fishing. And they traveled in winter using snowmobiles instead of dog-powered sleds.

Each substitution had a dual impact: it removed the need to use every part of the animals they hunted while at the same time steadily increasing their need for cash. In Gambell, for example, the transition to snowmobiles (called snow machines) over the past fifty years resulted in a decline in the number of sled dogs from five hundred in the 1950s to fifty to a hundred in 2008 (many of which are smaller breeds kept as pets).[2] These dogs had eaten large quantities of walrus meat, about 125 walrus per year, and their loss meant increased gas purchases to "feed" their replacements.

Because ivory had long been used to barter for what was not available locally, it was natural for Native Alaskans to turn to it as a source of money, especially when few other income options existed. Though

Ivory was always highly prized, its commercial value skyrocketed in the 1800s, when whalers killed thousands of walrus for their tusks. It became even more sought after in the early 1990s, when tourists, art collectors, and other consumers turned to it as an alternative for elephant ivory, whose commercial trade had been banned.[3] Demand from non-Native traders, who sold it to tourists and collectors, provided a ready market. While prices for raw walrus ivory vary according to quality, a pair of tusks can net $300 or more. In 2008, for example, several Internet businesses offered raw walrus ivory for $15 to $18 per ounce. Carved ivory commands a higher price, double the cost or more of the raw ivory depending on the quality of the workmanship, while complete skulls with tusk and lower jaw (measuring about 12 to 14 inches from front to back and weighing up to 20 pounds) can sell for between $1,500 and $2,500 each.[4] All anyone had to do to capture those profits was hunt the walrus and find a willing buyer.

Staring at the bloated body, Asigrook asked himself a difficult question: could his son or his peers be responsible?

The youth in his community were under enormous pressure. They didn't have the benefit he'd had of first living the old ways and then the modern ones. Asigrook had grown up with seal oil for light and heat, wearing hand-sewn seal and walrus-skin clothes, and eating Native foods (like walrus meat) caught by his family. His generation straddled

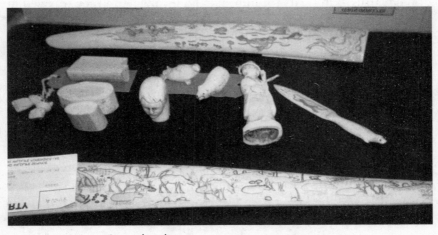

Carved walrus ivory. (Courtesy of Laurel A. Neme)

the two worlds, traditional and modern, and they knew enough to take the best of each while rejecting the parts that didn't fit who they were. His son's generation, however, had grown up in the modern world, and had not fully integrated the traditional ways into their psyche. They also wanted to escape their remote existence. Sometimes they did so with drugs and alcohol, like their peers in the lower forty-eight. Other times they did it by rejecting their cultural traditions and embracing everything modern. They were the first to depend on goods brought in from outside the island. As a result, they, like many non-Natives, relied less on the natural world for sustenance and often felt less respectful toward it.

An ambiguous legal environment that allowed nonwasteful hunting but failed to clearly define "wasteful" facilitated the transition from lack of respect to illegal killing. The legal vagueness combined with high ivory prices and the desire for cash created an irresistible lure for many, often in the younger generation but also among non-Natives, to get ivory by any means possible.

The sad result lay before Asigrook.

He got back on his four-wheeler and headed for home.

Headhunting had a high cost for the animals and the community, and its wastefulness went against everything his people believed in. It also spurred condemnation by environmentalists and animal rights activists, who called for elimination of the Native exemption in the Marine Mammal Protection Act. If they succeeded, it would take away the Natives' right to hunt—and end their way of life forever.

He and others in his community, especially the elders, had tried to address headhunting themselves. They'd imposed catch restrictions and punished violators. But the abhorrent practice continued. With such a strong pull for ivory from the outside world, they couldn't do it alone. They needed help.

In the fall of 1989, Al Crane squinted in the bright autumn sunshine. From the window of his small Cessna 185, he scanned the coastline of Alaska's remote Seward Peninsula, the westernmost point of the North American mainland. He grimaced at the scene below him—hundreds of walrus, almost all without their heads and tusks, had washed up on shore.

A special agent with the U.S. Fish and Wildlife Service, Crane was the first such officer to be stationed in northwestern Alaska (Nome).

He'd been hired away from Alaska's Fish and Wildlife Protection Division in 1974 to implement the newly passed federal Marine Mammal Protection Act, and he now had the unique arrangement of acting as supervisor, pilot, and field operative.

Crane had put a lot of effort into working with villagers on enforcement. In 1974, he'd launched an education campaign that included an extensive media effort in the three major local languages about how to comply with the law. His experience had taught him that to get compliance in this remote part of the world, the local people had to believe in the validity of the law and implement it themselves.

In Alaska, especially in the rugged terrain of the northwest, the "rules" for law enforcement were different from what was standard in the lower forty-eight states. Political realities meant that enforcement of laws, particularly those governing natural resources and Native subsistence, had to incorporate an understanding of the culture to have any chance of success. Hence, agents weren't able to disrupt age-old practices involving subsistence hunting without Native willingness and cooperation. Crane's posting in northwestern Alaska, the first of its kind for FWS, reflected the recognition of the need to work *with* the villagers, and he had done just that. In fact, he'd done so much that fellow officers accused him of being a social worker instead of a law enforcement officer.

Crane was tall and blond, but despite his different appearance, the Eskimos trusted him. His years in Alaska as a law enforcement officer, bush pilot, and devoted outdoorsman gave him a well-deserved reputation for approachability, fairness, and understanding of Native culture. That he was one of the early organizers of the Iditarod, and ran that grueling race in 1977, reinforced his credibility and toughness, which manifested in a natural, casual confidence and sense of forthrightness.

Crane knew the law needed to be enforced, but he also respected the Native position. In the Native view, the law, which allowed non-wasteful subsistence walrus hunting and required full use of the animal, hadn't caught up with the times and their changing needs. While ivory and meat were still valued, the shift away from sled dogs and walrus-skin boats as primary means of transportation meant they no longer needed as much meat or as many hides as they had previously. The law's failure to define "wasteful" implied that hunters had to use everything and leave nothing.

Crane agreed that it didn't make sense to require use of the *entire* animal when the community no longer needed every part. He thought the law should better reflect reality, and worked to define "wasteful" in a more appropriate way. Throughout his career, Crane fought to better incorporate the nuances of Native resource use into law enforcement activities. In the early 1990s, he drafted policy guidelines that specified exactly what hunters should bring back from each walrus they harvested, namely the heart, liver, flippers, chest skin with attached blubber (coak), some red meat, and the ivory. The dead walrus below him were one more example of the need for law enforcement to take this same careful approach.

Crane turned the Cessna westward and headed toward Cape Prince of Wales. Over the next few days he'd fly from village to village to meet with Native hunters and discuss the appalling sight below him.

Unfortunately, the slaughter was nothing new. After moving to Nome in 1974, Crane had flown the U.S. secretary of the interior (the agency that houses FWS), Cecil Andrus, on a tour along the coast and spotted over 350 headless walrus. Formal counts corroborated these observations. For example, in July 1975, 91 carcasses littered the beaches from Wales to Cape Espenberg, with most missing tusks. In September 1988, scientists counted 418 washed ashore from Wales to Barrow (for comparison purposes, 131 walrus were located between Wales and Cape Espenberg). Of these, less than one percent (0.72 percent) were intact with tusks. In August 1989, counts revealed 228 from Wales to Barrow (91 from Wales to Cape Espenberg). The widespread waste was both morally wrong and illegal. While Crane and Native Alaskans had tried to stop it over the past fifteen years, the scene kept repeating itself—carcass after headless carcass.

They needed to find a new approach.

Later in the fall of 1989, Crane sat in a folding chair near the front of the Gambell schoolroom. Meetings like this one between FWS and village hunters took place every spring to talk about the upcoming walrus hunt and every fall to discuss the harvest. As part of a long effort to improve relations between villagers and wildlife law enforcement officials and explain the intricacies of the relevant marine mammal protection laws, they gave Crane a chance to review the law and explain what FWS considered "wasteful" and hence illegal, to leave the main usable parts of the walrus, namely the hide, flippers, ribs, and other red meat. While these regular meetings now occurred under the auspices of the Eskimo Walrus Commission (EWC), an organization created in 1978 to represent Alaska's coastal walrus-hunting communities,[5] their amiable tenor demonstrated the hard-won trust the agent had cultivated with local communities.

At this meeting, as in others, local residents blamed Russian villagers, who hunted walrus on the other side of the Bering Strait, for the headless walrus that washed up on their shores. They claimed the Russians killed the animals and cut off their heads for the ivory, or else hunted them for subsistence but lost them during the hunt. Time and waves then brought the dead animals to the Alaskan beaches. If a carcas arrived still intact, Native hunters would take the tusks as the only part, aside from the rotten "stink meat" on the underside, that they could salvage from the decomposing bodies, or else beachcombers purposely flying their small aircraft would revel in the ivory treasure.

Crane listened to the explanations but doubted their validity. Native Alaskans did poach walrus, and a variety of casual conversations he'd had with villagers following other FWS-EWC meetings or informally on the street confirmed it. At a previous meeting in Wales, for example, a hunter had openly admitted headhunting because selling ivory was a ready source of cash and the quickest and easiest means to support his family.

Crane appreciated the pressures created by the cash economy yet thought them also a convenient excuse. Most Alaskan Natives would have agreed, even if they were reluctant to admit it. They scorned headhunting. It contradicted thousands of years of the tradition to use what they took and threatened the future political viability of subsistence hunting.

The meeting broke up and Crane rode back with his host, Tim Asigrook. The men remained silent until Asigrook brought up the past spring's poor harvest when, for the first time in twenty years, villagers had failed to catch as many walrus as usual. The Native hunter was worried that his people had brought a curse upon themselves by headhunting, and feared that, as retribution, the Bering Sea walrus might follow the path of the African elephant, "headhunted to near extinction by the very people who depended on them for their survival."[6]

Asigrook's worries had a basis in fact. Over the past 150 years, walrus hunting by non-Native whalers and commercial fishermen dramatically reduced their populations three times, with the most recent decline in the mid-1950s when numbers fell to just 50,000 to 100,000 animals.[7] While each time walrus populations were allowed to recover, the current level is unknown. The most recent survey, conducted almost twenty years ago in 1990, estimated the number at 200,000 animals.

Of that, subsistence walrus catches by indigenous Arctic people in Alaska and Russia average around 3,000 annually, a tiny fraction of the total. However, the actual number killed may be higher, with perhaps another 2,000 wounded and lost during the hunt and an unreported number poached solely for their tusks.

Nobody knows what level of hunting is sustainable. There are too many gaps in the information available, like the size of the population and the factors that affect it. The lack of data suggests that, by the time researchers detect a drop in walrus numbers, corrective measures could be too late.

Today, walrus are threatened by more than commercial exploitation. Global climate change has reduced both the extent and thickness of the pack ice, which means walrus have nowhere to rest or care for their young near good feeding grounds. Normally, walrus use their ice platforms as "taxis" to float closer to their all-you-can-eat buffet—that is, the nutrient-rich areas where they dive for clams and other crustaceans. When the ice pack is farther out, it ends up over water so deep that the animals cannot reach the sea floor to feed. The village of Wainwright, in northwest Alaska, provides a case in point. Throughout the 1990s, sea ice in August was normally 30 miles or less from the village coast. More recently, however, that distance has increased. Now it is typically more than 100 miles away, and in August 2007 it was 300 miles away resting over 1,500 feet of water—well over the 300-foot-or-less depth that walrus prefer for foraging.[8] The result, warned a team of researchers led by the University of Tennessee and including staff from the Woods Hole Oceanographic Institution, is that ice-associated marine mammals like walrus must adapt to raising their young in shallow waters without the benefit of sea ice for resting between dives. Otherwise, "a significant population decline of this species could occur."[9]

That concern was reflected in a February 2008 petition to FWS and subsequent lawsuit by the Center for Biological Diversity to protect Pacific walrus under the Endangered Species Act because of the likely consequences of global warming and offshore oil development. In May 2008, a similar petition and lawsuit resulted in polar bears being listed as threatened because of sea ice loss caused by global warming, the first time an animal has been protected because of global warming.

The impact of climate change on the walrus has deeper repercussions. Walrus play a major ecological role in their ocean ecosystem. They eat a huge amount, up to seven thousand bivalves, such as oysters and clams that live on the floor of the continental shelf, also called the benthic zone, a day. When they forage on the muddy bottom, they stir up the sediment, a process called bioturbation, which releases nutrients into the water and shifts organisms around to make them more accessible to others. In cold water, like the Arctic, organic matter such as algae tends to sink to the bottom rather than float closer to the surface as it does in warmer seas. Thus, walrus feeding habits affect the structure of sea life across thousands of square miles.[10] Consequently, a decline in their populations could hamper biological productivity across the Bering Sea.

Climate change and a drop in marine mammals also hurt Native Alaskans, who rely on their ocean "garden" for sustenance. For them, the sea ice acts "like a big conveyor belt"[11] to bring walrus and seals in closer range for hunting while at the same time making the ocean calmer for safer hunting. Without the ice, Native communities face shorter hunting seasons, larger swells, and more dangerous seas—and less chance of hunting success. In 2007, for example, Wainwright hunters harvested less than twenty walrus when normally they catch over a hundred.[12] At a time when traditional cultures are already under threat from other forces—like the transition into a modern cash economy—a decline in walrus populations adds yet another hazard.

Crane took Asigrook's fears seriously. He also recognized the conversation and others like it for what they were: unspoken and unusual requests for help. In the Native culture, leaders rarely went outside the community for assistance, preferring to solve problems themselves. A direct request for aid would have been improper because it would have been a serious breach of etiquette to put someone in the position of having to say no if they weren't able to help.

But Crane didn't want to say no. He understood that Native communities needed to navigate their own path on their own terms. If he could prove the headless walrus had been deliberately killed for their ivory, Native Alaskans would then have the ammunition to address the issue themselves.

The newly established U.S. Fish and Wildlife Service Forensics Laboratory was the perfect "munitions depot." Not long before, Crane had worked with the lab to prove illegal aerial wolf hunting in Alaska's Kanuti National Wildlife Refuge. While hunting in the refuge was legal, aerial hunting was not.[13] To determine criminal activity, the methods and means mattered, just as they did in this case. If anybody could determine how and why the walrus had died, the lab could.

In early 1990, Crane sat across from Goddard at an Anchorage restaurant and appealed for help. Crane's boss, Dave Purinton, assistant regional director of law enforcement, listened to the plea. His presence emphasized his support of the idea and the official, if unusual, nature of the request. The proposed investigation was atypical in that, generally, the lab's analysis connected a suspect to a crime. In this instance, however, FWS had no particular suspects. Rather, it simply wanted to know whether a crime had been committed.

Could the lab figure out if the headless walrus had died of natural causes, or been killed solely for their tusks?

Goddard was sympathetic. Several years earlier, in 1982, he had assisted undercover FWS agents in a raid of black market ivory traders in Anchorage. FWS agents had infiltrated an outlaw motorcycle gang that was illegally buying raw walrus tusks from Native Alaskans. The gang would send the raw tusks to Washington State, where Caucasian craftsmen carved "genuine" Eskimo figurines before shipping them back to Anchorage for the tourist market. The scheme flew in the face of the Marine Mammal Protection Act, which protected traditional Eskimo culture by letting only Native Alaskans own raw ivory. That act prohibited non-Natives from possessing the raw material (unless they found it on the beach and obtained a special permit from FWS), and allowed them only to buy and sell ivory when it was already worked by Native carvers. The fifteen-site raid had netted hundreds of tusks.

The Alaskan FWS request also built on the lab's first major success. One of the lab's chief scientists, Ed Espinoza, a brilliant Chilean-born criminalist, and his colleague, staff scientist Mary-Jacque Mann, had recently developed a method to distinguish modern elephant from mammoth ivory. Following the June 1989 CITES worldwide prohibition on commercial trade in African elephant ivory (commercial trade of ivory from Asian elephants was banned in 1976), traffickers falsified their documents to say their shipments contained ivory from ancient woolly mammoths, which was legal, instead of from modern elephants, which was not. Because mammoth ivory looks remarkably similar to that of elephants, the deception worked. Agents were powerless to stop them. That is, until five months later when the lab discovered a surefire way to tell them apart. After that, U.S. Customs officers and FWS wildlife inspectors could seize the smuggled elephant ivory.

Because ivory scams still frequently cropped up, examining the full spectrum of possible substitutes and also thwarting the illegal killing of other ivory-producing animals, such as the Pacific walrus, was an ongoing focus. The investigation of the headless walrus case would add to their knowledge of ivory, especially about how one of the main substitutes for elephant ivory was killed.

The walrus victims had died far from the reaches of law enforcement, probably on an ice floe miles from shore. Alaska FWS agents did not know where or why the animals died. Patrolling the vast expanse of ocean was an impossible task. Nobody but the hunters and the walrus knew what happened. But the walrus couldn't say and the hunters weren't talking.

It would be the lab's job to figure it out.

Normally, Goddard would have instructed Crane to send the corpses to the lab. But in this case practicality forced a new approach. Rather than ship one or more two-thousand-pound walrus carcasses back for examination, Goddard opted to send a team of forensic scientists—himself, ivory expert (and now deputy director) Espinoza, and the lab's chief veterinary medical examiner, Dick Stroud—to the crime scene.

Goddard was used to working out of a suitcase. He'd done it for the last ten years. Besides, it made sense to see the carcasses in situ because they could possibly pick up additional clues from the surrounding area.

But this case would be the first, and last, time the lab would go to a crime scene for such an extended time. Normally, for human murder cases, forensic scientists examine the physical evidence in their labs while crime scene investigators document, preserve, and collect those items and detectives use that information to identify the perpetrator and build a case for prosecution. In only rare instances of an especially serious or complicated crime scene will a forensics lab, given its backlog of cases and limited budget, send its scientists to the site.

This case, however, fit the bill. It was complicated, involving hundreds of victims scattered along a huge physical area. It was also serious. The situation had gone on year after year. Without scientific proof to negate Native Alaskan claims that they were scavenging already dead animals, and thus prove illegal activity, FWS was powerless to do anything.

In addition, this case was unique in that the question at hand was not whether one particular walrus had been killed illegally and who did it, but rather if a *pattern* of headhunting existed. Thus, the scientists needed to look at the washed-up walrus as a group. There was no way to preserve and ship dozens of walrus from their inaccessible beachcast spots to the lab.

Typically, the lab identifies the animal origin of wildlife pieces, parts, or products so that if those species are protected, the poacher or smuggler can be prosecuted for his or her crime. In this case, though, the victim was already known and the objective was not prosecution. It wasn't a matter of species identification, but a determination of illegal activity by proving the walrus had been killed wastefully. That would mean knowing more than the cause of death. It would mean discerning the intent of the hunters and the circumstances of their kills.

The lab had no established way to answer those questions. They would have to break new ground through trial and error to figure out an appropriate methodology.

To the forensic scientists, the carcasses would tell a story. They might reveal that the hunt happened in Alaska rather than on the Russian side, and thus negate the claims of "we didn't do it." They might also say that the animals *had* been killed solely for their tusks, and not simply lost during a legal subsistence hunt. That would definitively prove a problem existed and establish accountability. If Native communities didn't get a handle on headhunting, their entire right to hunt—and culture—would be even more threatened than it already was.

Too many walrus had died solely for their tusks. But could the lab prove it? And if they did, would either the Native Alaskans or FWS be able to stop it?

CHAPTER TWO

Walrus Forensic Investigation

How can a dead, headless walrus expose the intent of its killer?

That puzzle stumped the three scientists—Goddard, Espinoza, and Stroud—as they prepared for the walrus investigation. Because Native Alaskans hunt walrus in late spring and early summer, the scientists would trek to Alaska at the end of July, after the season's final storms, to examine that year's carcasses. But to make their trip worthwhile, they needed a way to answer the basic question: were the headless walrus killed solely for their tusks?

As in any case, they started with what they knew. Native hunters shot their prey at sea, either while the walrus rested on floes or swam in open water (a practice called pelagic hunting). Unless bad weather or other hazards prevented it, they butchered the animals on the ice and, if their intentions were for subsistence, took as much of the hide, meat, organs, blubber, and ivory as they could use.

Killing for subsistence was legal while killing for commercial purposes was not. Consequently, the scientists would focus primarily on why the animals died and use any information they could gather on cause or manner of death or on who did it, to point to the hunter's intent. They needed to establish whether walrus were being killed wastefully by Native hunters.

They would have little evidence to go on. Because the killings would have occurred somewhere at sea days or weeks earlier, before the animals washed up on shore, they would have no witnesses and no crime scene. Even if they had, wind and weather would likely have corrupted the physical or trace evidence. They would have to infer intent from the major piece of evidence they did have: the decomposing carcasses.

But what could a dead walrus tell them?

If the victim had been human, the scientists would have known what to expect. Regular crime labs use tried-and-true technology to produce results in which they know the chance for error. DNA testing in rape cases identifies suspects. Bullet trajectories and blood spatters reveal the position of the killer. But the wildlife crime lab was not so lucky. Nobody had worked with a walrus carcass before to ascertain whether it had been legally killed. They would have to adapt existing techniques and develop new ones to coax the walrus corpse into divulging everything it could.

During the winter and spring of 1990, in between their other duties, the scientists contemplated what data would signal wasteful kills versus subsistence kills. All three came at the problem from distinct professional viewpoints.

They began with Goddard's. Goddard's approach was determined by his background as both a cop and a criminalist. After graduating from the University of California–Riverside in 1968 with a bachelor of science in biochemistry, Goddard worked at the Riverside County Sheriff's Department as a deputy sheriff/criminalist. Ultimately he chose to focus exclusively on forensics. A charismatic, garrulous man with prematurely white hair and a coy white mustache, he went on to work at other crime labs before becoming the first director of the FWS crime lab in 1979. The wry twinkle in his eye and his humorous asides suggested that in his years of crime scene investigation he'd seen it all and was prepared for anything.

Criminalistics, Goddard's specialty, is a term often used interchangeably with forensic science. It refers to the examination, identification, and interpretation of physical evidence from a crime to reconstruct events and link a suspect to the victim. As Paul Kirk, the "father of criminalistics," noted, trace evidence "cannot perjure itself" or "be wholly absent."[1] Criminalistics is based on the theory that every contact leaves some residue in the form of evidence, such as blood, tissue, fingerprints, bullets, tire tracks, shoe impressions, or hair and clothing fibers.

The most obvious form of physical evidence they might reasonably uncover in the walrus carcasses would be bullets. Bullets could prove death by gunshot, reveal the type of rifle used, or even identify the specific weapon used in the hunt. That information might rule out Russians as responsible for the killings, and thus point to Native hunters. That would be a worthwhile discovery. However, their utility for indicating wastefulness was poor because guns were used by all hunters whether for subsistence or commercial purposes. The bullets wouldn't help them distinguish between the two. For that, they needed a better line of attack.

While Ed Espinoza was a criminalist like Goddard, he was also a skilled forensic chemist. He was a patient man, in his late thirties, with a crisp Chilean accent who spoke and acted in a deliberate way. He held a bachelor of science degree in medical technology from Loma Linda University in California, both a master's and doctorate in forensic science from the University of California–Berkeley, and had worked as an assistant professor of forensic sciences and as a private practice forensic consultant specializing in homicide cases before joining the lab in 1989.

Forensic chemists use highly specialized techniques to analyze the chemical composition of organic and inorganic substances such as poisons, fire accelerants, blood, tissue, and bones to determine how an organism died. They also study decomposition and weathering to infer what happened after death.

To prove wastefulness, the scientists needed to know what happened to the walrus after they died. If the walrus had been legally killed for subsistence, the carcass would lack not only the head but also other parts such as meat, hide, and flippers. If someone had severed the heads of already dead animals washed up on the beaches, it would indicate the also legal practice of beachcombing. If, however, the heads had been cut off before being beachcast, it could be a sign of illicit head-hunting.

Espinoza hypothesized that diatoms, microscopic (between 20 to 200 microns in diameter or length) single-celled photosynthesizing algae that live in both fresh and salt water, imbedded in the necks of the carcasses might tell them when the heads were removed—either before the dead animals entered the water or after they had washed up on the beach. Because living diatoms have specific salinity, temperature, and other environmental tolerances, species vary by location. Scientists then use this information to match the composition of diatoms in the victim's body to those in a particular water source. In human forensics, they are used in two main ways: to identify a specific body of water, like a lake, and to determine whether a victim died before or after entering water.

Scientists analyze diatoms in bodies recovered in water to tell if the body was alive or dead when it entered the water.[2] The theory behind this test is that if a person drowns, the diatoms in the water will reach the lungs and, if the heart is still beating, enter the bloodstream and circulate around the body, lodging in internal organs—kidneys, brain, bone marrow—before death. If the body was dead when it entered the water, diatoms would still reach the lungs through passive means, but they would be absent in the more distant organs because no circulatory transfer could occur.

The walrus situation was analogous. Although knowing if the animals were dead before entering the water was immaterial for determining headhunting, knowing if an otherwise intact carcass had its head removed before it entered the water *would* be a valuable indicator of wasteful hunting. If the head had been removed from an otherwise intact carcass on an ice floe before the body entered the water, there would be diatoms on the exposed neck area. If the head of an otherwise intact carcass had been removed after the body washed up on shore, there would be no diatoms present.

Espinoza did allow that waves splashing on the carcasses might leave diatoms, although perhaps not as many. For this method to be useful, the scientists would have to know how diatom concentrations and composition varied between the two scenarios. Yet that detailed level of diatom data simply wasn't available. They would need more research—and a lot of it. To acquire the information, the lab would have to extract diatoms from different water depths across the walrus's entire marine environment, purify them, and then analyze them. That would be a complex, expensive, and time-consuming procedure. They needed a better option.

The third member of the team, Dick Stroud, approached the determination of wasteful hunting from his medical examiner's perspective. Medical examiners—medical doctors with specialized training in forensic pathology—use their knowledge of disease and body processes to determine what caused a person's death. They perform autopsies and analyze organs, tissues, and bodily fluids for indications of the circumstances of sudden fatalities. Stroud, as a veterinary pathologist, was no different, except his subjects were animals.

Since his childhood in Texas, Stroud had always been interested in wildlife. An avid hunter and fisherman, he began his career in the early 1960s as a wildlife biologist collecting data from the fur seal harvest on

Alaska's Pribilof Islands, and then later participated in a pelagic research program where fur seals and other marine mammals were collected at sea and the stomach contents analyzed for species of prey. The dead animals never bothered him. To the contrary, he was used to working with animal carcasses in various stages of decomposition. To Stroud, the wonders of the functional body fascinated him and spurred his desire to study how the structure of an animal's organs and body systems changed due to disease, parasites, or injury.

Stroud returned to school and graduated in 1972 with a doctorate of veterinary medicine (DVM) from Washington State University. In 1978, while working at the Veterinary Diagnostic Laboratory at Oregon State University on stranded marine mammal carcasses from Oregon beaches, he completed the requirements for a master of science in veterinary pathology. He adapted what he learned on livestock and pets to wildlife in his pathology residency at the San Diego Zoological Society in 1980, and then joined FWS, where he worked first as a pathologist at the FWS National Wildlife Health laboratory in Madison, Wisconsin, and later as the coordinator for the Environmental Contaminants Program (investigating oil spills, superfund sites, and cyanide leach mining) at the FWS regional office in Portland, Oregon. In 1990, he transferred to the Wildlife Forensic Lab to become the senior medical examiner for wildlife, a position he has held for more than eighteen years.

From Stroud's perspective, the best way to tell if the headless walrus had been killed wastefully or for subsistence would be through a necropsy, or animal autopsy. For human victims, autopsies yield proof on the cause and manner of death, and whether the fatality was deliberate or accidental. Maybe the same process on the walrus could generate similar evidence—except it would be regarding hunting for subsistence or commercial purposes.

But how do you necropsy a walrus?

Stroud researched the process of walrus necropsies by talking with other wildlife veterinarians working on marine mammals, such as Sam Dover, a vet at Sea World, San Diego. Dover advised Stroud in the most expedient procedures for entering a walrus carcass and searching for signs of foul play. Yet even with this information, nobody had ever conducted a necropsy on a walrus for these purposes and under these conditions. It might not work. And still, none of the scientists had a clear idea as to how to deduce the hunter's intent from the carcasses.

By the end of May, the brainstorming and research had produced little in the way of a concrete procedure. Goddard and the others were frustrated, and it made no sense to proceed without some kind of plan. On June 4, 1990, Goddard wrote assistant regional director of law enforcement Dave Purinton suggesting the lab postpone its trip. The lab director explained that the research on diatoms had resulted in a "nonuseful technique," and that the only thing they could do in Alaska would be to dig for bullets, but that "there's no way to link the projectiles to the process of wasting the animal." Goddard recommended the forensic team wait until they could "come up with some other procedures that might help resolve the basic issues."[3]

The Alaska FWS agents rejected Goddard's proposal. They didn't want to wait another year, or longer, as hundreds more walrus died. They wanted to do something, and Goddard willingly agreed to send a team. But the team would treat this first expedition as a preliminary exploration into more promising methods.

In July 1990, the scientists prepared to leave. Espinoza flipped through his six-page checklist to see what supplies they still needed for the upcoming trip. He would lead the investigation, with Goddard helping to document and analyze the proceedings and Stroud running the necropsies.

In the corner of the lab's conference room, Stroud bent over several plastic storage bins, running a final check on the equipment. Staring intently from behind the large glasses that dominated his round, slightly freckled face, he focused on his task. A shy, quiet man, he wore jeans and a plaid flannel shirt that echoed the fifty years he had dedicated to living outdoors and working in nature. He had diligently investigated the gear he'd need to perform necropsies on the remote beaches of Alaska, knowing that once there, he'd have to make do with whatever he'd packed. Over the past weeks, he'd collected everything from extra-long knives to meat hooks, and even designed a special form with schematic diagrams of top, left-, and right-side views of walrus bodies and skeletons to record his findings.

Goddard poked his head into the staging area to offer assistance, but Espinoza had the situation well in hand.

Espinoza scrutinized the bins for the remaining items: metal detectors to locate bullets; guns and ammunition for unforeseen wildlife threats; and even industrial-strength soap and odor neutralizer. Given the stench emanating from live walrus, these last items would be vital for handling their dead and rotting bodies.

The scientists had mapped out a plan of action. They assumed they would find evidence of three scenarios. If the walrus had been killed for its tusks, only the tusks would be removed and the remainder of the carcass would have been left to sink and eventually drift ashore. They could identify these carcasses by the way the tusks had been removed and because the rest of the body remained intact. In the second scenario, when wounded and lost animals washed up on the beach, the scientists would likely find gunshot wounds with pathological changes indicating death sometime after being shot, as well as evidence of tusk removal after the carcass had been stranded. The recovery of bullets and location of bullet wounds would provide clues to hunting skill and techniques that might be used to identify illegal or wasteful activities. The third possibility would be natural mortality with recovery of tusks from the carcasses after they'd been cast on the beach.

With these hypotheses outlined, the team would start by counting the number of stranded walrus carcasses and comparing their observations with surveys from previous years. They would then fly to each carcass to examine it more closely.

They recognized that the carcasses might be too rotten for a meaningful postmortem evaluation. And even if they did find carcasses in adequate condition, they weren't sure if a necropsy would tell them what they needed to know. They'd have to be flexible to see what worked and what didn't. This trip would be only a starting point, aimed at establishing field protocols and identifying factors, such as the inability to reach each carcass, that would affect what they could do. Then, over the next three to five years, they hoped to develop a methodology and use it to ascertain if a pattern of illegal killing existed.

Everything was ready for this first trip. Now they just needed to wait for the last of the summer storms to deposit the victims on the beach.

In late July 1990, Goddard, Espinoza, and Stroud landed in Fairbanks after a ten-hour flight. Tired and rumpled, they walked to baggage claim where they found Al Crane and his subordinate FWS special agent Mark Webb, who would act as their guides. Crane stood with his

usual lanky confidence and greeted the scientists in his warm bari-
tone. Though Crane easily surpassed six feet in height, Webb was even
taller. A broad smile appeared beneath Webb's thick mustache as he
greeted the men. Though a relative newcomer who'd only lived in
Alaska for two years, he shared his boss's concern and enthusiasm for
the state's natural resources and the people who depended on them.
Crane and Webb would fly the scientists four hours north to the village
of Kotzebue, twenty-six miles above the Arctic Circle, in Crane's Cessna
185 and Webb's smaller Piper Supercub.

Kotzebue, situated on a narrow, three-mile-long spit of land on the
Baldwin Peninsula in Kotzebue Sound, was a relatively central launching point for the scientists to investigate the northwestern Alaska
beaches. As the gateway to four major but undeveloped national parks,
the Noatak National Preserve, Kobuk Valley National Park, Cape
Krusenstern National Monument, and the Selawik National Wildlife
Refuge, the area served as the home and breeding grounds for polar
bears, caribou, moose, black and brown bears, and millions of migrating waterfowl and shorebirds, while its offshore seas supported numerous sea mammals, including several varieties of whales, seals, and, of
course, walrus.

Kotzebue's coastal location at the confluence of three rivers also
made it a hub for ancient Arctic trading routes. When German lieu-
tenant Otto von Kotzebue "discovered" the area for Russia in 1816, he
found a large, well-established settlement and trading routes of Inupiat
Eskimos, who called the area Kikiktagruk, which means a place that is
shaped like a long island. Although weather makes the shipping season
brief—only one hundred days from early July to early October when
the sound is ice-free—Kotzebue still serves as a transfer point between
oceangoing and inland vessels, and with a thousand households, it is
one of Alaska's largest Eskimo villages, second only to Barrow. Like
many other northern Alaskan villages, its extreme remoteness means it
connects with the rest of the state only by air or sea. It has only twenty-
six miles of roads, attesting to the utility of airplanes and boats over
cars in this part of the world.

The scientists' first task was an aerial survey of Kotzebue Sound and
the southern Chukchi Sea to count walrus carcasses and plot their

locations. Once they had an accurate map of where the carcasses lay, they would return to as many as they could for closer examination.

Their route took them north along the coastal sections of the southern Chukchi Sea, from Cape Krusenstern up to Point Hope and Cape Lisburne, and then south and west, paralleling the exposed beaches and offshore barrier islands of the northern Bering Sea, and then to Topkok Head, east of Nome, an area home to 80 to 90 percent of the world's walrus. Throughout the length of their flight, the flat blue-gray ocean gave way to a skinny strip of tan-gray gravel beach that rose into an emerald and lime carpet of fragile tundra. Outlines of sunken polygons formed by the freezing and thawing of the ground divulged the shallowness of the vegetation, which sat upon endless permafrost.

As they flew, the drone of the plane reinforced the unchanging scenery's hypnotic effect, yet the scientists stayed alert by dutifully marking each carcass on their maps. The level uniformity of the landscape made spotting them easy, especially since Crane and Webb were flying low, and every ten or twenty minutes, they would glimpse one

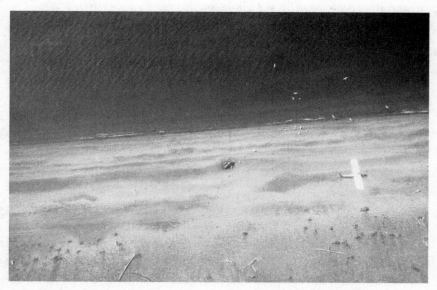

Walrus carcass from air. *(Courtesy of U.S. Fish and Wildlife Service Forensics Laboratory)*

and sometimes more. From above, the carcasses looked like large brown boulders, about the size and shape of a Volkswagen Beetle.

An hour into the flight the scientists sighted their first live walrus, a lone animal fretting on the rocky beach. The animal seemed reluctant to enter the water; it moved jerkily toward the ocean and then stopped and backed away. Its behavior was typical of a sick or injured walrus. When hurt, pinnipeds—marine animals with winged or finned (pinna) feet (pedis), such as walrus, seals, and sea lions—use up their blubber. Without this insulation, they become cold in the water, which prompts them to climb onto ice or shore to warm up and may make them unlikely to venture back in. If this walrus had been wounded by a hunter, it could fit the scientists' second scenario of animals wounded and lost (not immediately recovered) by the hunter. Measuring a carcass's fat layer could reveal if it was diseased or had been injured and forced into a situation similar to this one.

By the end of the day, the count totaled sixty-one substantially intact walrus carcasses, all with tusks removed, and four live walrus. While consistent with the number of walrus that Native hunters had reported they'd caught during that spring's hunting season, the count was lower than previous years. Two years earlier, in September 1988, an aerial survey covering a slightly different range (from Wales to Barrow) found over four hundred headless walrus. The decline wasn't necessarily due to less headhunting, however, but to the climate. Usually, the hunting season lasts from four to six weeks in spring depending on the weather, but during the past May and June strong southerly winds hastened the ice pack's retreat and gave hunters less time to harvest the walrus migrating along its edge.

Later that night, sleep was difficult because the scientists couldn't stop reviewing the day. They wondered why there were so many headless walrus. Maybe the next day's necropsies would tell them.

The following morning, the team loaded their gear and set out for the first carcass, located 12.8 miles southeast of Point Hope, about 200 miles from Kotzebue. At the site, the men emerged from the planes and the smell hit them hard. Goddard and Espinoza winced. While long inured to what might turn others' stomachs from working grisly homicides, the two scientists did not look forward to the next few hours. Stroud, however, was indifferent. He'd anticipated that the rotting carcasses would be "rather odiferous," but preferred to "do walrus than a baby diaper any day."

The long, narrow beach stretched endlessly in either direction. The scientists felt as if they had landed at the end of the world and, in a sense, they had. Far from human activity, nothing sounded but the gentle hum of insects and repeated slap of the ocean.

Aside from a sporadic piece of driftwood, the bloated russet carcass was the sole feature on the landscape. It lay fifty feet from the water's edge, where twenty-four hours of sunshine, which contributed to temperatures in the high 60 degrees Fahrenheit, had accelerated its decay. The bloated body bore little resemblance to a living walrus. Without its distinctive whiskered face and two-foot tusks, it appeared more like an enormous yet grotesque rubbery floor cushion with insect-infested gashes.

If the fatality had been a human, the methodology for figuring out how, when, and where the victim died, as well as who might have done it and why, would have been relatively straightforward. The procedures were well established, and one knew what to expect from the results. Yet wildlife forensics is still in the nascent stage where human forensic science was a century ago, and many cases are "firsts." For each new class of case, meaning one that involves a not-yet-submitted species of animal, part or product, the scientists must discover a procedure to resolve the issue at hand, be it identification of the species, cause of death, or another criminal question. After that, they must demonstrate that the protocol provides consistent results. Only then could they apply the methodology to the current investigation so that it would pass legal muster.

Stroud had pointers from other marine mammal veterinarians, and he himself had dissected his own share of seals. But this case was unique. It would be the first time a medical examiner performed a walrus necropsy in a remote setting to determine wastefulness. That made it unlike any other walrus dissection.

Their first order of business was to determine an exact timeline of how a dead walrus rotted in this unique climate, and if a badly decayed carcass would yield clues about the types of weapons used and the hunting practices. Bone-weathering patterns could indicate the time of and conditions after death, but they also had to establish how the Arctic water affected the erosion of a walrus skeleton. Information about where the killing might have occurred, using drift trajectories, could also prove useful. Finally, they'd need to research both the conditions under which a dead walrus would float and how wind, waves, and currents influenced when and where it washed ashore. The only way to find out was to dig in.

The three men donned yellow coveralls and Stroud began the procedure as he would any necropsy, whether in the field or in the lab: with the carcass's history. He asked himself the standard questions: What circumstances surrounded its discovery? How long had it been there? What weather conditions might have manipulated it?

The carcass rested on its right side. Two small logs, which had probably been used to pry the posterior over so that someone could cut out its penis bone, lay near its hindquarters. Male walrus lack an externally visible penis. They hold their organ inside until ready to reproduce, at which time they extend it using a twenty-inch bone called a baculum (or oosik). Like other aspects of their biology, such as a small head with no external ear flaps, this trait streamlines their bodies and better adapts them for swimming and conserving heat. The walrus baculum is highly sought after and commands significant commercial value,[4] perhaps because it is the longest of any living mammal.[5] Someone had not only removed the baculum from this carcass but had also chopped the tusks out of their front sockets, leaving a bloody mess.

Randomly scattered holes pockmarked the walrus's back. Stroud examined them more closely and found that several had bruising around the punctures that distinguished them from the other holes. These were almost certainly bullet wounds.

He searched for a pattern of shot placement. If he found more wounds in the lower and back part of the animal, it might indicate that the animal had been shot while still in the water—evidence of pelagic hunting. Pelagic hunting is a highly wasteful and inefficient method for harvesting meat, skin, or other parts because shots fired from a low platform, like a boat, at a marine mammal surfacing for air tend to result in "gut shots." While ultimately fatal, gut shots don't kill the animal right away. When the dead walrus finally does drift ashore, the only usable parts remaining are the tusks and stink meat (on the underside of the body). While the bullet wound placement alone wouldn't indicate pelagic hunting, if the hunters had also failed to remove meat, it could mean that their only desire was to kill for ivory. In contrast, if Stroud found more shots in the head and neck, it would indicate that the walrus had been killed while out of the water, the method preferred by subsistence hunters because it allowed them to harvest the animal's parts.

Espinoza waved the metal detector over the possible gunshot wounds. If they could find the bullets, they might not only identify the rifles and ammunition and individual hunters but also establish the types of hunting practices that wounded rather than killed walrus. As they soon discovered, however, finding a bullet in a walrus was no easy feat. The detector hummed steadily, apparently operating well, but gave no sign of the presence of metal. If Stroud had been at the lab, X-rays of the carcass could have quickly led him to the foreign objects. But on an isolated beach 2,400 miles from the lab's X-ray machine, the only way would be a manual search.

Stroud slipped on rubber gloves and grasped the thick wooden handle of his seven-foot-long flensing knife. Positioning the two-foot blade on the walrus's back close to its neck, he braced himself with one foot on the animal's back and the other on the ground and sliced downward. With short, controlled strokes, he split the tough one-and-a-half-inch hide to reveal a hand-sized layer of gray blubber underneath.

The stench, already unbearable, actually worsened. Stroud showed no sign he smelled the stink but Crane and Webb blanched and turned away, as if to busy themselves with the aircraft. The two agents were happy to leave the science to the scientists. Goddard and Espinoza could hardly breathe either. But they had no choice but to persevere.

Dissecting a walrus carcass is cumbersome and tricky. The tough hide is heavy, with one flipper weighing up to 150 pounds, making slicing it an arduous task. Stroud straddled the carcass to cut through the six-inch layer of fat and grayish-pink-and-brown muscle below. Espinoza acted as surgical nurse by holding back the skin with large hay hooks and metal stakes and leaning his own body back to provide a counterforce to Stroud. Goddard, having capitalized on his position as lab director to snag the easiest job for himself, was happily snapping pictures to document each step of the necropsy.

To make the carcass more manageable, Stroud carved out chunks and set them aside. He didn't have to worry about preserving the body as he would have if it had been human. The hard work dulled his blade, forcing him to stop every fifteen to twenty minutes to sharpen it.

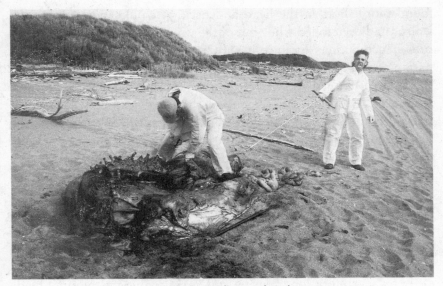

Veterinary pathologist Dick Stroud and ivory expert
and chemist Ed Espinoza dissecting a headless walrus carcass.
(Courtesy of U.S. Fish and Wildlife Service Forensics Laboratory)

While he did that, Espinoza waved the metal detector over the lumps of muscle and fat laid out on the beach. But he still found nothing.

Stroud turned to the rib cage—a good location for potential gunshot evidence—and switched to long-handled pruning shears, the kind used for small tree branches, to clip away at some of the rib bones and remove part of the chest wall. Bloody fluid seeped out, and he opened the chest cavity more so that he and Espinoza could bail it out and look inside. The men scooped out cup after cup of fluid until they had filled a five-gallon plastic bucket and drained the cavity.

Stroud slid his flashlight systematically over each section, hoping to confirm bullet wounds, but after all the careful excavation, all he found was fibrous coagulated blood adhering to the lining. Stroud noted that the fibrin tags adhering to the surfaces of the thoracic cavity indicated that the animal probably died sometime after it was wounded.[6]

Undaunted, Stroud continued the necropsy. He switched to a smaller butcher knife with a heavy high-carbon molybdenum steel blade and detached the organs. Once more, he laid the pieces—this time the heart, liver, and kidneys—in a line on the sand and Espinoza passed the metal detector over them. Again, nothing. Espinoza kept at it but no amount of scanning changed the result.

They repeated the process all morning and into the afternoon, but five hours after they began, they gave up trying to find a bullet in this carcass. The scientists flipped off the metal detector and, a few minutes later, Goddard's camera stopped clicking, intensifying the quiet of this distant stretch of coast. There was nothing left to do. Stroud had gone over every inch of the carcass. The necropsy was finished.

While frustrated, the three men refused to concede defeat. Instead, they chalked up the experience as information to employ in the future. They had learned the mechanics of a walrus necropsy. They also had an appreciation of the challenge of unearthing a two-and-a-half-inch or less fragment of metal in a two-thousand-or-more-pound hippo-sized mass.

Yet their prize—a method to determine wasteful hunting from walrus remains—eluded them. This victim had probably been struck and lost, not headhunted. Perhaps the next carcass would have been killed illegally. And maybe, just maybe, it would tell them something.

With dozens of dead walrus ahead, the scientists moved on to their next victim, less than a half mile southeast. This walrus's head had been severed, leaving sharp, almost surgical, knife cuts on the cartilage between the cervical, or neck, vertebrae. Somebody had wanted the tusks and knew how to get them. But was it the main reason for this animal's death?

A huge hole pierced the walrus's abdomen on its left side going through the thick blubber and stopping just short of the peritoneal cavity. Stroud looked for the cause of death. He measured the blubber, but the animal had adequate fat deposits, so poor health wasn't the issue. Instead, signs of internal hemorrhaging suggested that gunshots had caused the large, gaping wound. Stroud tried to confirm this hypothesis but once again he couldn't find any bullets or bullet tracks.

They found their third carcass a half mile away. This walrus lay on its belly high on the beach. Stroud examined the body, slicing methodically through each layer, as Espinoza assisted and Goddard recorded the process with his camera. While the head of this carcass remained intact, someone had slipped the tusks out of their sockets, probably after decomposition had expanded the skull and loosened the tight fit. Numerous holes punctured the walrus's back and left side, and intestines protruded from one of the wounds. All of these signs again pointed to death by gunshot, yet clear evidence of bullets continued to elude the scientists.

The lack of bullets disappointed the scientists. While still not able to prove intent, they might at least match bullets to a type of weapon. That data could point to hunters on one side of the Strait, and either prove or disprove which group—Alaskan or Russian—had killed the beachcast, headless walrus. Yet the failure didn't faze them. It only meant they'd have to take a new approach.

Weary and covered in muck, the scientists cleaned up their tools, repacked their equipment, and headed back to camp.

The following day, August 1, 1990, the men flew to another carcass they'd plotted on their map—this one located about an hour northwest from Kotzebue, near Point Hope. The soft ground forced them to land on the far side of an Arctic stream from the victim. Unfortunately, in trying to ferry the men and equipment across the hazardous terrain, the Supercub's landing gear collapsed. Forced to scrap the examination, Webb stayed with the disabled plane to wait for a mechanic while Crane and the scientists flew back to Nome to find new transportation.

For the pilot/agents, the delay was simply part of a day's work in Alaska's perilous environment. But for the scientists it was yet another constraint on what they could hope to accomplish. Every protocol they came up with had to be reliable and replicable. In addition to the challenge of digging around a massive, badly decayed carcass, walrus necropsies presented the dual drawbacks of inaccessible locations and transportation glitches that were standard in this part of the world.

Was there a better way?

After switching to an old mail truck, Crane chauffeured the three scientists about twenty miles north of Nome toward three carcasses they had spotted during their aerial survey. With no roads and little suspension, the short distance stretched into hours of bumping and jarring. The drive ended unexpectedly when their squat green-and-white four-wheel-drive jeep got stuck in another Arctic stream.

Reaching the walrus carcasses to perform necropsies was proving more and more difficult. The goal of examining all sixty-one carcasses was starting to look nearly impossible.

While the expedition was meant as a preliminary assessment, the complications were making it apparent that necropsies might not be feasible or productive. The three necropsies thus far had failed to locate bullets despite signs of gunshots, and they had not exposed definitive evidence that differentiated between walrus hunted for subsistence and those killed for their tusks.

Often, the wildlife lab's scientists staggered up promising but faulty paths before finally finding one that worked. For example, in trying to uncover a method to distinguish between elephant and mammoth ivory, Espinoza and Mann searched for variations in hardness, density, and the amount of fat, and even discovered that very old samples fluoresced under ultraviolet light. Yet that method failed whenever the outside layer of ivory had been removed. To find a process that worked under all conditions, they examined over 10,000 pieces of ivory before homing in on the fine, curved lines radiating out from the center sections of the tusks and discovering that the angles formed by these intersecting dentinal tubules were always greater than 110 degrees in modern elephant ivory and always less than 90 degrees in ivory from mammoths.

Setbacks were a standard part of wildlife forensics, and these scientists were used to the seeming lack of progress. Dead ends taught them what didn't work, and that knowledge was just as important as learning what would. It was a normal part of scientific discovery.

With their jeep stuck, Crane and the scientists set off on foot and found the first of the next set of carcasses easily enough. While from the air it had looked like a headless walrus, on closer inspection it turned out to be a seal, so they kept going. Their next victim, located about ten miles west-northwest of Nome, had been reduced to fifty pounds of unrecognizable meat, most likely by bears and other scavengers. Espinoza scanned what he could with the detector but located no bullet fragments. Too little remained for any other type of postmortem exam.

About five miles farther, they reached the next carcass, their fifth. This was clearly a walrus, but a disgusting one. The entire head had been severed from the body and holes punctured its back. Thousands of maggots swarmed the tissue in its neck and had dissolved it into a greasy glutinous mess. The insects had partially skeletonized (eaten the tissues attached to the bones) the cervical vertebrae, which now poked through what remained of the jellylike neck. The bones were picked clean, as if they'd been there for a long time, but strangely, the rest of the body exhibited a much earlier stage of decomposition.

Stroud began dissecting the carcass while Espinoza tried to locate a bullet. The metal detector chirped over and over, as if urging the scientists to keep searching. Stroud complied and dug through the bloody mass until, finally, he had nowhere else to look. Disappointed, they gave up. Stroud hypothesized that the persistent chirping occurred because fragments had come off the main bullet as it mushroomed, while the butt or main portion traveled deep into the carcass where they could not locate it. They were so close and yet *still* so far.

The men walked on and, a few miles farther, located their next target. As they got within a few meters, they recognized the shapely tail of a whale. With their latest failure fresh in his mind, Goddard proposed an experiment. They could use the dead whale to test both the metal detector and their techniques for recovering a bullet and find out once and for all if their gear actually worked on a marine mammal.

Goddard took out his .357 and fired two rounds: one into the ground, as a control, and a second into the whale carcass. Espinoza waved the detector over the sand and quickly located the first shot. Then he passed the instrument over the whale, concentrating on the entrance wound and the bullet's likely path. Nothing. But since there was no exit hole, the second shot *had* to be somewhere inside. The experiment had proved what they had already decided—the metal detector wasn't working as they'd hoped.

Disheartened, they called it a day. Thinking of the tasks that lay ahead, they walked up the shore to get away from the smell and stopped for the night. If the detector couldn't pick up a lead bullet in blubber four to six inches thick, to have any chance of finding a bullet, they'd have to cut the carcasses into much thinner pieces and lay them flat on the beach before using the detector.

The next day, their last in the field, they were guided to their final carcass by its stench. This huge decaying mass reeked far worse than the others. To make matters worse, it was riddled with gaping holes and open sores. Crane walked away in disgust. Even though he'd worked around hundreds of dead walrus, this one topped the charts.

The carcass lay on its left side, about fifty feet from the water and several hundred yards from an inhabited house. Someone had chopped out the tusks from the thick frontal bones of the skull, and bone fragments still stuck to the tissue. Black burn marks charred its skin and muscle and covered its back. Clearly, someone had tried without success to dispose of the smelly carcass by burning it.

Stroud, Espinoza, and Goddard pulled on coveralls, rubber boots, and gloves to ready themselves for the necropsy. Beginning his visual exam of the body, Stroud discovered two bruised holes on the right side of the neck. Espinoza ran the metal detector over the spots but, unsurprisingly, found nothing. Even so, Stroud thought the holes might be from bullets. He inserted two arm-length aluminum rods into the holes to track the bullets' possible course. With a little effort, he slid the probes along what seemed to be clear projectile paths until they stopped, about six to ten inches beneath the hide.

Stroud picked up a narrow, six-inch knife and carefully sliced the muscle along the track of the first rod until, at last, he hit something solid. Keeping his knife steady, he inserted his gloved hand into the tissue to meet the blade and felt around so as not to lose touch with the

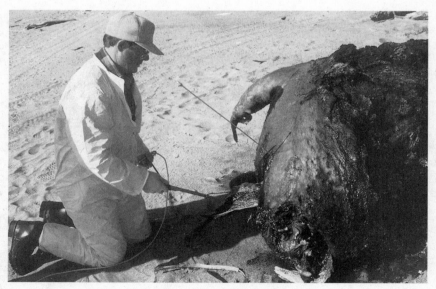

Veterinary pathologist Dick Stroud tracing bullet path in walrus carcass.
(Courtesy of U.S. Fish and Wildlife Service Forensics Laboratory)

object. Moments later, his face lit up. He pulled his hand out from the muscle and held up his prize: a small metal fragment and several flakes.

The men grinned at each other and placed the items in an evidence bag, which they marked and sealed for later analysis. Encouraged, Stroud sliced along the second path. When he was about six inches in, he grinned again. He slipped forceps in to meet his hand and pulled out a large-caliber bullet.

Basking in the small victory, Stroud thought about the location of the bullets. While these injuries clearly caused bleeding, he did not know if they were immediately fatal and figured there must be additional wounds elsewhere. He opened the thoracic cavity and siphoned out ten gallons of bloody liquid. The lungs and heart appeared intact and he found nothing amiss. He cut through the abdominal cavity and bailed out another five gallons of red fluid. Traces of intestine floated in the bloody drainage, suggesting the walrus had been shot through the bowel. Inch by inch, Stroud inspected the abdominal wall with a flashlight but saw nothing that suggested gunshots. He searched with the metal detector but could discern no additional signs of bullets or damage.

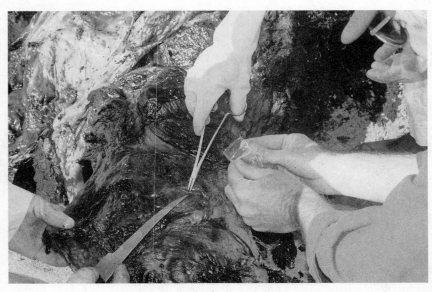

Cutting out bullet from walrus carcass.
(Courtesy of U.S. Fish and Wildlife Service Forensics Laboratory)

Finished, Stroud collected his tools while Goddard and Espinoza soaked the carcass with gasoline and set it on fire. A few minutes later, the flame changed from bright orange to deep red-orange and then blue as the carcass smoldered and blistered.

Their investigation had been both a success and a failure. They had encountered carcasses from a range of scenarios, some shot, lost, and then beachcombed and others possibly poached for their ivory. They'd learned to dissect a decaying walrus, and they'd learned the limits of their metal detector. But they still had no definitive way of telling whether a particular walrus had died from ivory poaching.

The necropsies, although clearly a necessary first step, had yielded less than expected, and finding bullets turned out to be far more complicated than they'd anticipated. Most important, however, they'd discovered the difficulties of operating in that remote environment and the constraints on what they could accomplish. Just *getting* to each carcass was an ordeal, and with the incomplete answers from the necropsies themselves, continuing full dissections of individual carcasses was not a feasible option. Before they could do more, the scientists would have to return to the lab and see what else their expedition and the evidence they had recovered would reveal.

Back at the FWS wildlife forensics lab in Ashland, Oregon, during the fall of 1990, the scientists hoped the hard-won bullet they'd found would provide some answers as to who had done the killing: Alaskan or Russian hunters.

After talking with the team, Mike Scanlan, the lab's ballistics expert, analyzed the bullet under his optical comparison microscope. Using his Fowler Dial caliper, he measured the diameter, or caliber, of the bullet, then counted the lands, or cuts into the bullet, and grooves. He noted how the land impressions angled from the tip to the back, indicating the direction of twist, and then measured the width between each of the lands and grooves.

Scanlan compared his data to the Federal Bureau of Investigation's General Rifling Characteristics File that was established and updated by its Firearms-Toolmarks Unit and determined that the bullet was a .284-caliber copper-jacketed projectile. But he couldn't tell for sure what type of weapon had fired it. The best he could do was narrow the possibilities to a 7mm Remington Magnum cartridge fired from an

Alpine Sporter, Remington Model 700, or a Tikka M65 rifle, or a 7x61 mm S&H fired from a Schultz and Larson M60. Despite this uncertainty, the information proved useful. Neither of these bullets was used by Russian hunters, who favored steel-jacketed bullets; the copper ones were preferred by Native Alaskans. This slug pointed straight to Alaskan hunters.

The scientists were pleased with the finding but still needed more proof. Espinoza had a hunch that the location of the carcass could shed light on who had beheaded it and dumped it into the sea. Despite a boundaryless ocean, the Russian and Native Alaskan communities hunted in relatively distinct areas. Two of the Alaskan subsistence hunting regions were located north of St. Lawrence Island and a third was east of Little Diomede Island. If Espinoza could show that ocean currents could only have carried the dead walrus from these Alaskan hunting grounds to their final resting places on the Alaskan beaches of the northern Bering Strait and southern Chukchi Sea, then he could disprove the claim that those carcasses had been killed on the Russian side.

Subsistence hunters used their knowledge of ocean currents to find their cryptic kills, walrus wounded during the hunt that died later, after they'd been cast on the beach. He would do the same thing but in reverse.

Espinoza considered the aerial survey map they'd made during their trip and compared it to charts showing ocean currents, wind patterns, and community hunting areas. He then reviewed thermal images from NASA and located three main currents through the Bering Strait: one from the Yukon River that hugged the Alaskan coast; a second through the middle that moved north from the Pacific; and a third, noticeably warmer, that came from China and followed the Russian shore. With these general bearings, Espinoza set out to find hard data on where the dead walrus would drift.

To simulate the walrus' movements, he turned to three drift experiments that had been done in the same geographic area. In the first, completed over thirty years earlier for the U.S. Office of Naval Research and the U.S. Atomic Energy Commission,[7] sixteen hundred bottles were released at thirty-five stations in the northern Bering and southeastern Chukchi Seas and their paths were analyzed. In the second, conducted in 1979 for Alaska's Department of Fish and Game, scientists had evaluated the movement of a possible spill from a proposed oil and gas lease sale in the Norton Basin. The third, a field test run in 1990 for the U.S. Department of the Interior's Minerals Management Service (MMS), had also mimicked pollution drift trajectories by following satellite-tracked surface buoys. These studies gave Espinoza a good idea of where a floating object would end up.

But would a dead walrus even float?

Research published in the mid-1970s by renowned marine mammalogist and walrus expert Francis H. "Bud" Fay, as well as the personal experience of Special Agent Crane, told Espinoza that if a walrus carcass was cut open, which would happen during subsistence hunting, it would sink and stay sunk. Knowing this, poachers would sometimes slit a walrus's belly to hide the wastefulness of their kill. However, if a walrus carcass was relatively intact, it would sink initially but later rise, perhaps in two to three days, as putrefaction of the tissues, especially in the stomach, intestines, and abdominal or thoracic cavities, produced enough gas. Once the carcass was buoyant, the wind, waves, and currents would bring it to shore.

Confident that a walrus carcass would follow the same patterns as the bottle drift trajectory studies, Espinoza predicted that in the two hunting areas north of St. Lawrence Island, circular surface currents would bring dead animals back to the island, while those wounded in the third area, east of Little Diomede Island, would drift either toward the northern shore of the Seward Peninsula along the coastline from Cape Prince of Wales to Cape Espenberg, or to the western Alaska shore from Cape Krusenstern to Point Hope.

He examined additional data, including National Oceanic and Atmospheric Administration (NOAA) maps on distribution of currents and the known movement of lumber down the Yukon River, which deposited in Cape Prince of Wales, and confirmed his calculations. The headless walrus on the beaches of Alaska's Seward Peninsula could not possibly have been killed in Russian hunting areas.

So far, all the evidence—shot placement, the bullet they'd found, and walrus buoyancy and drift patterns—suggested wasteful and illegal hunting practices. But they needed much more evidence before Crane and the Native communities could do something about it. They had to prove that a pattern existed.

But how? They needed a method more practical and efficient than individual necropsies to determine whether or not a dead walrus was killed for its tusks.

Espinoza examined the photographs from the necropsies. As he inspected the images of bloated bodies, the stark whiteness of the severed vertebrae peeking out from the bloody tissue of the walrus' necks caught his eye the same way it had in the field. The appearance of the vertebrae was odd, almost as if someone had cleaned them.

He flipped through the remaining pictures. Even though the clean, white neck bones looked weathered, the skin's reddish-white color pointed toward an earlier stage of decomposition. But the disparity couldn't be possible: how could rates of decay vary within a single carcass?

Like any organic object, dead walrus rot in an orderly sequence: first stiffening and bloating; then popping and deflating when an external force, perhaps a seagull picking at the flesh, pierces it and lets the gases escape. After the flesh disintegrates, some tissue clings to the bones and they stay black until microorganisms, wind, and sun eventually clear the remaining tissue and bleach them white. Arctic weather influences the time frame of decomposition, with warm, wet summers allowing the carcass to complete this cycle in as little as two weeks and cold temperatures disrupting it for up to a year.

No matter the variation in lengths of decay, many of the beached carcasses examined in Alaska didn't fit the sequence. Instead, they exhibited two separate stages of decomposition: the bodies were more or less intact, mostly at the "popped" stage, but the exposed vertebrae in the neck were already white. Espinoza was determined to find out why.

When Espinoza told his butcher he needed nine fresh, partly fleshed articulated cow leg bones, with joints still connected by tissue and ligaments, the man, used to the scientist's odd requests, barely blinked before gathering them in several plastic bags. Espinoza took them back to the office and set them on his black lab table next to the ax, handsaw, and chain saw he'd laid out for his experiment—he planned to replicate the weathering patterns he'd seen on the walrus's vertebrae. He'd start by using the three implements to create three types of cuts that simulated the hunters' methods. He'd then take the bones to the Oregon coast to see what happened when they were subjected to water and weather.

Espinoza grasped the first cow joint firmly and chipped at it with short, sharp strokes of his ax. The jagged edge grew as bone chips flew across the table. He repeated the procedure on two more bones. Then he switched to the handsaw, slicing back and forth to cut the ends off of three more joints, leaving dust particles in his wake. Finally, he slipped on clear plastic safety goggles and positioned the remaining joints in a vise. The chain saw's sharp whirr roared through the lab as he gently touched the teeth to the samples. At the moment of contact, its pitch rose irritatingly until, seconds later, he finished. He turned it off and ran his index finger across the edge of the cut. Smooth. Much more so than the previous sets.

With a hand drill, he bored holes through each bone. He then threaded thin nylon cord through the openings and knotted it around the samples. For one bone of each set, he added a second rope, attached to a heavy rock. Preparations complete, he was ready for his bone-weathering experiment. He repackaged the joints and put them in the refrigerator.

The next morning, with the bones packed in a couple of plastic coolers, he drove two hours to a U.S. Coast Guard station at Oregon's Gold Beach, where the experiment would begin in earnest. He would put the cow bone samples in three different microenvironments— marine subsurface, tidal, and partly vegetated rocky beach—to simulate the exposure of the neck bones.

Espinoza lugged one of the coolers to the nearby pier, waded into the water, and pulled the cooler along as it floated next to him. He fastened one bone from each set to the pylons so the tide would lap over them when it came in.

He carried the second cooler high onto the beach, away from the tideline. There, he hammered a metal stake into the grassy sand and secured the next set of bones. They'd be exposed to the sun and salty mist but remain untouched by the ocean water.

Next, using a Coast Guard boat, he tied the last set to a buoy floating about fifty yards from shore. He tossed the bones and their attached rocks overboard, knowing they'd stay underwater.

Now all he had to do was wait.

Thirty-five days later, eager to see the results, he returned to retrieve the bones. Back at the lab, a cursory visual exam showed clear variations among the bones. Dark brown oily splotches stained the tidal samples, perhaps because of some tissue residue. The beach bones, too, had blood and tissue remnants, but unlike the tidal ones, they appeared white and dry underneath. Only the fully submerged set looked anything like the exposed vertebrae he'd seen in Alaska and which stood out in the photos: white and clean of residue. Now he knew. The walrus vertebrae must have been exposed in the salt water for some time *before* landing on the beach.

Espinoza wondered why marine scavengers and microorganisms would feed only on the neck, and not on other parts of the skeleton, too. The only explanation was that the walrus' heads were removed at the time they were killed and before they drifted to shore. *If* the results of Espinoza's bone experiment held for the severe Alaskan waters, and *if* a carcass exhibited no other evidence of subsistence harvesting, the forensics lab would have an indisputable and efficient way to tell whether or not a particular walrus died because of ivory poaching.

Sitting in his Fairbanks office during the summer of 1991, Webb opened the FedEx package containing new sets of Espinoza's carefully prepared cow joints. He shook his head and stroked his dark mustache as he examined them. This was not a typical special delivery. Crane had assigned Webb to assist Espinoza in a scaled-down investigation of more walrus carcasses, and Espinoza would arrive in less than a month. First, Webb would fly up to Nome to begin the bone-weathering experiment in the Arctic waters of the Bering Sea. Webb had been planning to go north anyway for his regular preseason meetings with Native Alaskans; he'd add this testing to his to-do list.

When he got to Nome, Webb drove to the rocky pier at the edge of town and, carrying one of the plastic coolers, picked his way over the huge boulders until he was far enough out. He threw the first set of bones into the water and watched as they sank beneath the weight of the rocks he'd attached. He then tied the other end of the rope to metal stakes hammered into the boulders. They'd stay put.

He knotted the second set to the pier where the bones would be intermittently submerged. Carrying the third cooler, he strode up to the ruby sands beach, away from the sea, hammered a stake into the ground, and secured the third group of bones to it.

Nineteen days later, Espinoza arrived. He and Webb drove from the Nome airport to retrieve the bones before flying out to the northwest beaches to begin the exams. As soon as they pulled the bones up from the pier, Espinoza saw that these samples exhibited the same patterns as his Oregon experiment, confirming his conclusions and validating the proposed methodology for this, his second expedition.

The two men planned to fly the coast between Cape Espenberg and Cape Prince of Wales and look at every dead walrus they found using a new approach. Instead of doing a full necropsy on each carcass, Espinoza would concentrate on the presence or absence of three things: evidence of harvesting meat or parts other than ivory; unusual bone weathering; and the method of tusk removal. Skilled Native hunters detach a walrus's head by cutting at the atlantal-occipital junction, located about a foot behind the neck. A walrus head does not end where its neck does; its skull cap continues for twelve more inches. Cutting the head at the junction is the quickest and easiest method and leaves behind a clean, surgical cut. Inept hunters or beachcombers chop out the tusks, leaving a bloody mess of severe cuts and hatchet marks to the face and jaw (maxillary structure) of the walrus. Alternatively, tusks pulled out with minimal effort indicate the skull's prolonged exposure to water, which causes the bone to expand, and is a sign the carcass washed ashore intact. Together, these three features would constitute proof of wasteful hunting.

The next day, they flew from Nome to Cape Prince of Wales and then traveled northeast until they spotted their first carcass. They landed without trouble a short distance from the walrus and didn't bother to unload. This wouldn't take long.

Webb placed a crime scene marker on top of the body and Espinoza snapped a few pictures. The scientist walked around the animal, clipboard in hand, and marked the GPS (global positioning system) location on his worksheet. Then he scrutinized the condition of the skin, surface blubber layers, putrid smell, and scavenger activity and estimated the stage of overall decomposition of the carcass. The white cervical vertebrae poked out where the head should have been, contrasting sharply with the rest of the decay. On the underside of the walrus's belly, cuts indicated that someone had tried and failed to make the body sink. Espinoza jotted down his findings and shot more photos as illustration. Thirty minutes later, they got back in the plane and moved on to the next scene.

They flew from carcass to carcass along the desolate Alaskan coastline, stopping once to refuel near an equipment cache Webb had set up earlier. At each carcass, they duplicated their documentation of the animal's condition. Each time they repeated the process, the more adept they became. Working as a team, they eventually took as little as fifteen minutes to gather the data required. At about seven p.m., with the sun only slightly lower in the sky, they flew back to their campsite.

After several more days of gathering data, they had documented 105 carcasses from Point Hope to Cape Prince of Wales, a huge increase over the 61 carcasses the scientists had counted in their first week-long trip, which surveyed a longer strip of coastline from Cape Lisburne, 40 miles northeast of Point Hope, to Topkok, located about 120 miles southwest of Cape Prince of Wales past Nome.

Espinoza flew back to Oregon to analyze the evidence. For each carcass, he had three key facts:

1. The condition of the exposed cervical vertebrae—if the head had been removed, were they bleached or stained?
2. The way the hunter had removed the head—was it via a surgical cut at the atlantal-occipital junction, where the lower part of the back of the skull meets the top of the first cervical vertebra, or via chopping?
3. The presence or absence of meat harvesting—had hunters taken any meat or just the tusks?

Using this information, Espinoza put each carcass into one of five categories:

- Category I—headless carcass with clean cut at neck and exposed white neck bones
- Category II—head intact but tusks removed
- Category III—headless carcass with severe cuts and exposed oily, blotchy neck bones
- Category IV—fully intact carcass
- Category V—carcass too rotten to examine

The first group contained carcasses with vertebrae separated at the joints. This meant a skilled hunter had removed the head in a clean, surgical manner at the atlantal-occipital junction, thus exposing the neck bones, which now appeared white and clean of tissue or cartilage. Unless the hunter also took some meat, flippers, or other traditionally harvested parts, the headless walrus in this category represented purposely wasteful and illegal hunting.

None of the other scenarios confirmed unlawful harvesting. Carcasses found with their heads intact but their tusks pulled out with minimal effort—Category II—indicated legal harvest of the tusks of walrus that had died from either natural or man-made causes and then washed ashore intact. Walrus in the third category, with tusks chopped out and oily and blotchy cervical bones, also pointed to legal harvest of tusks by beachcombers after the carcass had been cast on the beach with head attached. Fully intact carcasses, in Category IV, had either died naturally or been shot and never recovered, while Category V contained walrus carcasses too rotten to examine. Their advanced decomposition—indicated by the gray-white color of their skin, caving in of the abdominal cavity, decayed flippers, exposed rib bone, and disarticulation (separation of joints)—made it impossible for Espinoza to infer anything.

Finally, after eighteen months of considering the problem, Espinoza had the evidence he needed. He could establish a pattern of illegal hunting.

Because the locations covered by earlier surveys diverged from one another, the scientist focused on the area of commonality, the 150-mile or so stretch of coast on the northwestern side of the Seward Peninsula, to assess trends. For purposes of comparison with previous aerial surveys of beachcast walrus, Espinoza concentrated solely on the 70 carcasses located between Cape Prince of Wales (near the village of Wales, the westernmost point of the North American continent) and Cape Espenberg, just north of the Arctic Circle in the Bering Land Bridge Natural Preserve.

Of the 70 carcasses he'd just examined there, about 75 percent fell into the first category—headless with a surgical cut and bleached neck bones. Within this group, 85 percent (44 carcasses) exhibited no attempt to recover anything other than the ivory. No meat, no organs, no flippers. Espinoza concluded that these walrus had been killed only for their tusks. But more than that, he'd established a straightforward approach to determine scientifically whether or not a walrus had been wastefully and illegally killed.

During the summers of 1992 and 1993, Espinoza returned to Alaska to count and examine more beachcast walrus with Webb and a third agent, Kim Speckman. Finally, he had enough evidence to establish a broad pattern of headhunting. Over the three summers, Espinoza had found 102 headless carcasses with a clean cut and exposed neck bones with no meat harvested, which confirmed poaching. While the exact percentage of headhunted carcasses declined over the course of the investigation, with 85 percent found in 1991, 53 percent in 1992, and 23 percent in 1993,[8] the results proved that Native Alaskan hunters were killing walrus for commercial, not just subsistence, purposes.

After more than four years of hard work, the lab's results confirmed what Native Alaskans and FWS agents already knew: walrus *were* being headhunted for their ivory. The lab's findings eliminated excuses and provided an opening for FWS and Native communities to work together for change.

CHAPTER THREE

Native Alaskan Solutions
to Walrus Headhunting

At the time of the lab's investigation, the scientists didn't know that their work was running parallel to a separate undercover operation by FWS into the ivory black market and ivory-for-drugs trade. In 1989, when Native leaders solicited FWS's help with headhunting, which led to the lab's inquiry, they also sought help for what they saw as a driving force behind the corruption of their youth: cash for luxury consumer goods and drugs, and illicit ivory as the source. While the resulting investigations were separate, the two crimes—illegal selling in the ivory black market and illegal hunting in the form of headhunting—were intimately related. Much of the illicitly traded raw ivory likely came from illegally killed walrus, and the carcasses of those poached animals were the same ones the lab examined.

FWS launched Operation Whiteout in April 1990, just a few months before the lab's first Alaska expedition. The initiation of what would become a three-year covert investigation into the ivory black market stemmed, in part, from the opportunity presented by the April 1989 arrest and October sentencing of a non-Native Gambell man (married to a Native woman) for trading drugs, money, and rifles to rural Native Alaskans for their raw walrus ivory. In exchange for a reduced sentence, he gave FWS agents an "in" to the closed circles of black market trading and helped two FWS special agents, Robert Standish and George Morrison, establish themselves as wholesale traders of raw ivory and Native handicrafts. The agents worked from a phony Anchorage storefront and traveled frequently with their informant on buying trips to remote villages.

Although the scientists were unaware of the sting, the lab's research altered it significantly. After the first year of both investigations, the scientists' initially inconclusive results prompted Morrison and Standish to expand the focus of their operation. After reading the lab's August 1990 preliminary report, Morrison took to heart its call for "additional investigations into the actual hunting practices . . . to confirm the assumptions made here on pelagic hunting of walrus . . . [and] to document the wastefulness of this practice."[1] Every time someone walked through the door of their fake warehouse, the agents suspected that the raw ivory came from an illegal headhunt, but the only way to know for sure would be to catch poachers in the act. The Operation Whiteout agents would do just that. They would extend the focus of their investigation from solely illicit sales to the source of their products: wasteful hunting.

Proving wasteful hunting wouldn't be easy. The lab's analysis had already encountered multiple obstacles in making that determination from the headless carcasses. It would be equally difficult in the field because wastefulness was relative. Many diverse circumstances, such as an impending storm, could force hunters to take only a small part of the animal—for example, the tusks. In those cases, leaving most of the animal wouldn't be wasteful, it would be smart. To prove illegal poaching, Morrison would have to be on the boat to see what happened and gauge the circumstances himself. For that, he'd need to con a poacher into taking him on a hunt.

In June 1991, Morrison's opportunity arrived. He was on one of his regular undercover ivory-buying trips in Diomede, a small village of 150 people located on the western side of Little Diomede, an island three miles from Siberia in the Bering Sea. The agent had planned to continue to Wales, the next village on his itinerary, but bad weather had forced the only commercial transportation, a weekly helicopter, to cancel its flight.

Morrison used the delay to his advantage and asked a local boat captain, Glenn Iyahuk, if he could buy a ride to Wales the next time he went walrus hunting. To the agent, the captain was a potential suspect for wasteful hunting. Morrison had watched Iyahuk and his crew take turns selecting trophies from a pile of sixty walrus heads after returning from other hunting trips. And a few days earlier, he had seen him return from a hunt with fourteen walrus heads, six hearts, two flippers, and two livers—not what Morrison would have called a legal and nonwasteful subsistence harvest.

After days of hearing about Morrison's travel woes, which were both genuine and a pretext to join the hunting crew, Iyahuk agreed to bring him along as soon as the weather changed. Hoping to put together concrete evidence, the agent offered to videotape the hunt and give Iyahuk a copy. Iyahuk agreed, perhaps because he was proud of his hunting ability and welcomed the prospect of pictures. However, the boat captain said he couldn't guarantee Morrison would make it the thirty-five miles to Wales because hunts and weather were always unpredictable.

A few days later, the weather cleared enough to go out for walrus. Iyahuk waved Morrison over as the agent left the Diomede post office to tell him. Though it was seven-thirty in the evening, the sun was still high in the mid-June sky. With twenty-four hours of daylight, Iyahuk would depart shortly. An hour later, Morrison climbed into the hunter's thirty-foot skinboat, which was already loaded with rifles, radios, and food, and quickly took his seat in the middle among the dozen people in the crew, which included two teenagers. Boys are typically introduced to hunting at an early age, around six or seven. James Brooks, former commissioner of Alaska's Department of Fish and Game, recounted in his book, *North to Wolf Country*, that when Iyahuk was young, the boy had cried when his father and other hunters first told him to shoot a walrus calf in the head and he couldn't do it. By the end of the season, however, the boy had witnessed enough killing that his sensitivity had dulled.[2] Out of necessity in his world, he'd gained the dispassionate attitude necessary to allow him to shoot the walrus.

The helmsman guided the boat carefully through the ice, searching the sky for dark patches on the low-scudding clouds—signs of open water pockets and possible routes to the walrus. Despite the walrus' large size, finding them in the ocean's broad expanse isn't easy. The hunters had waited days for the right combination of weather, wind, ice, and seas, well aware that poor conditions could easily turn their venture into a tragedy. Each had known hunters in their village who had died during hunts. In addition, the climatic shifts that had thinned the ice, prompting the animals to arrive earlier and leave sooner than in the past, gave every hunt an extra sense of urgency.

After several hours, they heard the distinctive bell tones, knocking, and tapping of walrus in the distance. The helmsman navigated slowly through the ice chunks toward a group of about a hundred walrus huddled on a large floe. As the men got out and inched toward the animals,

Morrison positioned himself behind them on a ridge of ice, where he'd have a good view. He turned on the camera and pointed it at the hunters.

When they'd crept close to the walrus, the men stopped. Bracing themselves on the rocking floe, some standing and others kneeling, the hunters raised their guns and, almost on cue, began shooting. One after another, shots rang out and the seemingly slow, complacent animals bleated alarms and bumped and shoved each other in a race to the sea. Unlike seals, which drag their hind ends around, walrus can "walk" on all fours and sprint on land as fast as a person can run.

A young, roaring bull lunged into the water and lifted its head, its strong herd instinct triggering its defense of the others. But Iyahuk and his crew kept firing, first at the walrus on the floe and then at the ones in the water. Anything that moved was fair game.

If this had been a traditional subsistence hunt, the hunters would have aimed only at the walrus still on the ice, which would be easier to retrieve. They also would have tried to avoid those in the water, though that wasn't always easy in the melee, and aimed at the third crease at the back of the walrus' necks—the surest spot for a quick, clean kill. They wouldn't have wanted the animals to suffer.

But these hunters didn't care.

Two minutes later, the frenzy of shooting stopped. All the targets were either dead or gone. Morrison kept the camera running and walked closer, watching the hunters head straight to the animals on the ice. They ignored the ones in the water and didn't even try to recover them before they sank.

Iyahuk approached one dead walrus, took out his knife, removed the head in a surgical swipe at the atlantal-occipital junction, and set it aside. He slit into the belly and looped a rope through the opening so that his men could pull the large animal onto its side. Then he cut again, removing the oosik, or penis bone.

There was no doubt in Morrison's mind now. These hunters had one objective: to get the commercially valuable parts of the walrus.

Morrison kept his expression neutral even though he abhorred the waste. Killing these marvelously awkward and ugly mammals solely for their tusks was criminal, but he couldn't stop what he saw in front of him. To interfere in the middle of the vast and inaccessible Bering Sea, alone with the hunters and guns, would have been suicidal, and it would have compromised his other cases. Besides, he'd get his chance later.

Morrison put the still-running camera down on the ice next to him and tried not to be obvious about recording. When the men had finished, they rolled the largely intact animal over the edge of the ice. As the dead walrus sank in the dark water, the hunters moved on to their next victim.

In February 1992, while the lab was planning its third Alaska excursion to test its protocol for determining wastefulness from carcasses, the covert part of Operation Whiteout closed and the next stage began. Although snow hindered the takedown, federal agents seized over 700 pounds of walrus ivory and charged twenty-nine people with illegally selling and buying ivory.[3] Those charged included Native hunters, among them Iyahuk and Asigrook's son,[4] as well as non-Native traders in Nome and Anchorage. The sting touched almost everybody in northwestern Alaska—from St. Lawrence Island to Diomede to the mainland—and would reverberate in the communities for years to come.

After FWS had revealed Operation Whiteout in February 1992 and played the bloody hunt video at its press conference, national media attention (including a piece on *Dateline*) ignited an intense debate about walrus hunting.

Throughout Alaska, matters related to subsistence use of natural resources, especially when conflicting with law enforcement, always generated deep passions and fears that Native rights would be taken away. In this instance, while they detested wasteful hunting, Native Alaskans worried that Operation Whiteout and the gory reality of headhunting as vividly revealed in the undercover film would trigger a backlash against lawful and nonwasteful subsistence hunting.

The most controversial of the Operation Whiteout–related trials came in July 1992 against Iyahuk and four of his crew. The hunters had been charged with three counts of failing to harvest meat from ten walrus, their total take from the all-night June 1991 hunt that Morrison recorded, and one count of conspiracy to violate the Marine Mammal Protection Act. Natives and non-Natives packed the second-floor room of the U.S. District Court in Anchorage, an expression of the intense interest in this case. After Morrison testified and walked the jury through the video step-by-step, lawyers for the defense argued that Iyahuk and his crew behaved rationally. The defense claimed that it made sense to shoot as many walrus on the ice as they could, and then fire into the water to kill wounded ones, to deter survivors from attacking.[5]

The defense lawyers then took an unusual turn and admitted the hunters wasted the walrus, but said their actions were justified because the meat was contaminated with toxic pollution and inedible.[6] Despite living in a pristine and remote area, the meat and blubber of walrus and other marine mammals can contain toxic substances, including pesticides, industrial chemicals like polychlorinated biphenyls (PCBs), and mercury, deposited by air in the Arctic. The Eskimos, at the top of the Arctic food chain, bore the brunt of that pollution when they ate the tainted meat. The defense maintained that the Diomede hunters on trial *couldn't* have wasted something that was *already* garbage.[7]

The line of reasoning resonated with people in the courtroom. The traditional way of life was already under attack from the transition into a cash economy and the increasing influence of the outside world. Just as the demand for ivory from non-Natives provided an incentive for poaching, contamination of Native foods by industries located well beyond the isolated villages evoked sympathy for the challenges of balancing traditional and modern ways of living.

The prosecution took care to recognize the legitimacy of this concern.[8] To have credibility in this venue, it needed to demonstrate its sensitivity to the Native situation, and it did so by refocusing attention on the real issue: what the hunting method said about the hunters' intent. Hunting practices, *not just edibility,* determined wastefulness. In this case, the men ate walrus meat for lunch while out on the ice, proving toxins weren't a concern, and they'd shot at walrus in the water without even *trying* to retrieve them.

Benjamin Nageak, a Native leader from Barrow and chairman of the Eskimo Walrus Commission,[9] agreed. His appearance on the stand represented a turning point in the case in both the relationship between Native Alaskans and law enforcement, and in the fight against walrus poaching more generally. Nageak explained that Native hunters are taught at a young age not to waste the resource: they must retrieve the walrus they shot or wounded. The lack of any attempt at retrieval by Iyahuk and his crew, he said, "was contrary to what [he] was taught."[10]

In the courtroom, the silence after Nageak's testimony was palpable.

Never before had a Native Alaskan leader spoken out against one of his own in public. His willingness to do so gave other Native Alaskans "permission" to speak out, too, and the courage to do so. His choice defined a new era that signaled Native intolerance of wasteful walrus hunting and implicitly indicated Eskimo willingness to cooperate more closely with FWS on law enforcement in the future.

A couple of days later, the jury found Iyahuk and four of his crew guilty and, three months later, the crew were sentenced: Iyahuk to ten months in prison, the others for two to six months.

The lab's scientists, who had been purposely kept in the dark about Operation Whiteout so as to maintain their neutrality, welcomed the confirmation of what they had found in the field. Only rarely did they receive separate verification that they had gotten the crime scene right.

By October 1992, of twenty-nine defendants charged as a result of Operation Whiteout, twenty-five were deemed guilty by plea agreements or trials; charges were dismissed on the other four. Penalties ranged up to a maximum amount of $6,500, and one person was given eighteen months' jail time.[11] The proportion of beachcast carcasses wastefully killed, as measured by the wildlife forensic lab's aerial surveys, declined from about 85 percent in 1991 to less than 25 percent in 1993.

The prosecution team, along with an expanding circle of Native leaders, celebrated the outcomes. Rather than being defeats for hunting, they saw them as victories that would allow the subsistence ethic to continue.

Yet the Operation Whiteout prosecutions were a double-edged sword. While they abhorred wasteful hunting and illegal ivory sales, Native Alaskans worried about the possible fallout: public opinion turning against subsistence hunting altogether. Debates regarding the reauthorization of the Marine Mammal Protection Act, which contained the exemption that allowed them to hunt, were about to start, with congressional hearings scheduled in 1993. Native Alaskans tried to stanch potential negative consequences from Operation Whiteout with a statement that demonstrated their loathing of wasteful take. In October 1992, the Eskimo Walrus Commission unanimously passed a resolution urging all Native hunters to take only the walrus they needed and to comply with all provisions of the Marine Mammal Protection Act. Meanwhile, FWS continued to educate the public about the law through a series of meetings that discussed plans for random spot checks of returning hunters to enforce marking, tagging, and reporting regulations. The agency also reiterated its intent to prosecute those who took only ivory.

With such high stakes, a delicate balancing act by Native leaders began to bolster the legitimacy of subsistence hunting while downplaying the pervasiveness of lawbreakers. Nageak, whose eloquence symbolized a major shift in the Native position, tried to place the Operation Whiteout court cases in a broader perspective. "The vast majority of the people who use marine mammals do so in a non-wasteful manner and will continue to do so indefinitely," he said.[12] "The use of these resources is important to the indigenous people . . . and 99.9 percent of them would not do anything which would disrupt or hurt their continued use of these resources. As in most societies, there are those who do not follow the laws of the land and they are the ones who get the most attention, and unfortunately those of us who are law abiding citizens get lumped in with them. We must do our best to make sure that those who break the laws are reported and they go through the court system as most people do when they break the laws."[13]

The arguments would resonate in Congress. In 1994, the Marine Mammal Protection Act was reauthorized and the Native exemption was retained. Yet shifting the blame to a few "bad apples" stunted a more comprehensive approach to wasteful hunting. The lab's results, still more than a year away, would change that tendency by exposing the wider-spread nature of the problem.

In June 1994, the lab presented its findings to Arctic hunters directly when Goddard and Espinoza flew with FWS special agent Webb to Point Hope, a small Inupiaq subsistence-hunting community of 750 residents[14] located 150 miles north of the Arctic Circle and recognized as the oldest continuously inhabited community in all of North America.[15] Their boots crunched on the soft spring snow as they entered the conference room where a dozen or so members of the Eskimo Walrus Commission waited.

At the gathering, the scientists explained how bleached cervical vertebrae, white and free of visible organic matter, could be combined with evidence to show that the hunter took no meat, indicating that the animal was killed illegally, only for its tusks.

The proof was convincing. Nobody at the meeting disputed the scientists' conclusions.

After the meeting, at a celebration of the first successful whale hunt of the year, one of the hunters stood before Espinoza as the scientist contemplated his *muktuk* (whale skin with blubber that resembled a watermelon cube).

"We knew," the man said, referring to the lab's findings. "We just didn't know if *you* knew."

Taking a page from the Eskimo's handbook, Espinoza nodded and gave no hint of the smile inside. The lab had done its job. It had applied crime scene techniques, evaluated evidence, and answered the question it had been asked: had the headless walrus been hunted legally for subsistence or wastefully for only their ivory?

The investigation would have a dual impact. Because of the difficulties its scientists had encountered, in the future the lab would forgo extensive field investigations because of the drain on its limited manpower. Three senior scientists had been in the field for eight days for the first excursion, and one had been gone for weeklong periods over the next three years. Given the backlog of evidence awaiting analysis, the lab determined that its limited manpower would be more efficiently spent applying their skills evaluating evidence at its Ashland lab. Since its walrus work, the lab has had many opportunities to go to crime scenes, most recently in May 2008 to evaluate the death of six endangered sea lions killed below the Bonneville Dam, which links the states of Washington and Oregon, in open traps aimed at stopping them from eating Columbia River salmon, which are even more endangered than the sea lions. But rather than go to the site, the staff opted to conduct X-ray examinations at the lab,[16] and they have embarked on limiting field crime scene investigations to a day or so since Espinoza's last visit to Alaska in 1993.

For the Eskimo communities, the lab's results would play a role in reorienting their approach to wasteful hunting. Because of their results, nobody could hide behind finger-pointing or bogus claims of salvaging already wasted walrus, and Native Alaskans were pressed to take more comprehensive action.

● ● ●

Over the next couple of years, FWS and the Eskimo Walrus Commission tenuously collaborated to curb walrus poaching. Yet their
approaches differed. FWS concentrated on law enforcement while the
Eskimo Walrus Commission preferred to educate hunters. The opposing perspectives made the relationship between the two uneasy, and
despite initial signs of hope and change after Operation Whiteout
and release of the lab's results, illegal hunting remained a "hot button"
issue.

In the spring of 1996, the situation came to a head when some
Native hunters reported large groups of exploded walrus washed up
throughout the Arctic northwest: almost thirty on Punuk Island east of
St. Lawrence Island in late May; twenty on drifting ice near Sledge
Island off Nome's coast a week later; and more on the floes between
Diomede and St. Lawrence Island.[17] Those who reported the carcasses
hated the waste and wanted FWS to help address it.[18]

To get a handle on the extent of the problem, Webb, who had
taken the now-retired Crane's job, and a colleague surveyed the area to
count the total number of headless walrus. Buzzing in the Supercub,
Webb tried to emulate the lab's procedure, although from the air and
without landing. When he spotted their first carcass along the shore
from Kotzebue to Shishmaref, he circled the plane in a long, slow arc
to get a better look. He noticed flashes of white bone shining through
the almost black muscle. He jotted down the approximate location
and continued farther down the coast. With each sighting, he repeated
the process.

The results were disturbing. All told, they'd counted over 160 headless carcasses. When the results were published, media and public
interest in the FWS probe grew. Providing updates and responding to
journalists' questions, Webb and other FWS officials explained that
hunters' reports of large numbers of headless carcasses appearing
after a storm prompted their investigation.

In response, Native leaders and other Kotzebue hunters insisted that
the dead walrus, particularly those washed up in Kotzebue Sound, had
either died of natural causes, been killed outside the region, or been
shot by local hunters and subsequently lost. Then, when they drifted
into the area, beachcombers took the ivory.

The refrain was a familiar one, and Webb disputed these claims
publicly in the newspaper. He'd seen the intact bodies with white bones

where the heads should've been, and he knew what they meant from his years of working with Espinoza. Focusing on the seventy headless carcasses in Kotzebue Sound, Webb alleged "those animals just didn't drift in"[19] but were killed the previous spring on the pack ice, where hunters removed the heads and then dumped the headless bodies into the sea. But Webb wasn't a forensic scientist and didn't have the credibility of an impartial observer. That opened the door for Native Alaskans and others to dispute his assessment.

Brendan Kelly, a research associate at the University of Alaska–Fairbanks and a close colleague of respected walrus expert Dr. Francis "Bud" Fay, expressed concern that the headless walrus found that year were "assumed to be the result of head-hunting without a proper investigation."[20] To him, that meant a full necropsy like the ones the lab had done during the first summer of its investigation. As tensions rose, an editorial in the *Anchorage Daily News* called on the FWS to "do its part by performing necropsies on beached walrus carcasses."[21] The NANA Regional Elders Council of the Northwest Arctic Borough echoed the demand, saying FWS should "reserve judgment about the cause of death without proper necropsies on the dead walrus"[22] and complaining that the agency "branded the Northwest Arctic Native community as poachers without a thorough and complete investigation."[23]

A forensic examination of the carcasses would have given everyone involved a better idea of how many were legally or illegally beheaded. And because the lab's assessment would have been independent and unbiased, it would have taken the friction out of the public discourse and allowed all the parties to focus on the real issue: walrus poaching.

Yet nobody asked the lab to investigate.

Because Webb had the procedural knowledge to assess the carcasses, FWS likely saw no need to bring the lab in. It would add no new information. And it would not have led to identification of suspects. But in the highly charged cultural milieu of northwest Alaska, it was a missed opportunity. A neutral, scientific assessment could have alleviated tensions, refocused attention on wasteful hunting, and improved the working relationship between FWS and Native Alaskans. That, in turn, would have been good for the walrus.

Instead, hostility grew. Because they feared Webb's statements might give animal rights activists the fuel they needed to stop subsistence hunting altogether, the agent quickly became a target of Native

Alaskans' animosity, and the situation was exacerbated by his handling of an unrelated situation in Kobuk.[24]

Chuck Greene, mayor of the Northwest Arctic Borough, said, "The early media reports unfairly tagged all Native hunters with allegations of waste and poaching. Later reports attempted to correct the mistake, but the impression will be left in some minds that ALL Natives hunt illegally. As government officials, we all need to be aware that our allegations can be used to fan the flames of prejudice."[25]

Similarly, Caleb Pungowiyi, director of the EWC, noted that "deliberate misinformation and disinformation . . . concerning native hunting and efforts to stop all hunting . . . will be devastating to our native community."[26]

In response to the allegations and to show that not all Native hunters were wasteful, Native groups, from the Eskimo Walrus Commission to the Indigenous People's Council for Marine Mammals, called for Webb's resignation.

"EWC commissioners ask for the resignation of Mr. Mark Webb based on the conduct of his investigations and his accusations of wasteful hunting through the media prior to any indictments or convictions of any persons. We take this matter very seriously and hope that you will at least conduct an investigation of his conduct in order to avoid further deterioration of the relationship with the native community," Pungowiyi wrote in a letter to David Allen, FWS regional director.[27]

In this politically charged environment, defusing the situation was critical. While forensic exams might have stopped the arguments about whether what they'd found at Kotzebwe Sound was headhunting and led the conversation back to the issue of stopping wasteful hunting, the time for that had passed.

But the agency couldn't fire Webb.

"The allegations against him do not warrant such action," FWS Regional Director Allen replied.[28] Webb was just doing his job.

Yet the agency had to do something to reduce the bitterness. FWS needed to work *with* the Native communities. The ocean was simply too vast for it to patrol. The only way it could enforce the law was with the support of the people. For this situation, FWS viewed Webb's approach as too "black and white" and his way of expressing his observations too emphatic. Consequently, the agency forced Webb to transfer out of Alaska in early 1997. Not what Webb wanted, but he had no choice.

Hostilities eased. Both sides wanted to avoid future problems. For its part, FWS agreed that when it had no specific suspect, it would consult the Eskimo Walrus Commission before investigating a headhunting case. It also promised to include EWC members on aerial surveys done as part of those inquiries. At the same time, the EWC pledged to report anyone suspected of illegally hunting marine mammals and also to step up self-regulation efforts in the communities.[29]

"We're all working toward the same end," said Dave McGillivary, FWS supervisor for marine mammal management in Alaska. "But there are people out there who aren't on board and some of them may never be."[30]

There would always be lawbreakers; the issue was how to reduce the number. The lab's investigation was a good start. It put the issue squarely on the table. It confirmed the crime and identified the culprits as Native Alaskan hunters.

But the lab's analysis was not part of a broader criminal process. Unlike most of its other cases, this one involved no particular suspect and could not result in an indictment. While its results had increased awareness, it could not force change. Native communities would have to do that themselves.

As with subsistence communities around the world, to end wasteful hunting, Native Alaskans would have to change their attitudes. They would have to *want* it to stop.

Over the next eight years, the Eskimo Walrus Commission, elders, and other Native hunters pursued a variety of tactics to shift mind-sets toward nonwasteful walrus harvests. Many focused on giving young people a better appreciation of traditional hunting methods and values to slow down headhunting. In Kivalina, elders had monthly meetings with the village's young people "to discuss traditions and . . . teach [them] not to waste."[31] With modern equipment such as guns and motors making it easy to kill large numbers of walrus and feasible to harvest only their commercially valuable parts, elders believed teaching the younger generation their traditional conservation values was a good way to ensure that the animals would not be wasted.

"These younger hunters, when they go out there, they get as many as they can. That is no good. We need to only take what we need," Shishmaref hunter Harvey Pootoogooluk articulated.[32] "The way our young people are hunting now . . . they'll shoot at anything and don't even bother to go hook it or whatever. I think that needs to change," Shishmaref hunter Davis Sockpick complained.[33] Diomede hunter Herbert Milligrock concurred, explaining, "These young guys don't know. . . . When they get excited, they shoot any old way."[34] Another Diomede hunter, Charles Menadelook, advised that "experience is the best teacher. When you make mistakes, they stay with you. And if you have someone knowledgeable to correct you, that's even better."[35]

But elders were dying, and taking the old ways with them.

"Our elder count is way down," Wales hunter Luther Komonaseak noted.[36]

Old-timers provide a quality of memory that guided life in this harsh, unforgiving environment. Their loss was like knocking "down a thousand-acre stand of mature timber";[37] it irrevocably changed the place and the culture.

The communities needed to capture their knowledge before nobody was left who cared about walrus for anything other than their tusks. To do that, the Eskimo Walrus Commission initiated several documentation projects to record traditional ways. Through a video project that started in 2004, Native villagers filmed the long-practiced and nonwasteful hunting methods in Gambell, Savoonga, and Diomede, the three main walrus-hunting villages. With funding from the FWS, the EWC bought equipment, trained local people as videographers, and set up subcommittees in the villages to edit the content.

"Something is missing among our young people," explained Vera Metcalf, Eskimo Walrus Commission director since 2002.[38] The video would express the spiritual aspect of why these communities hunted. The reason was more than just to eat. Hunting brought them back to nature and reconnected them with their ancestors. As a people, they respected nature, and respected conservation methods. By getting back to their roots through the videos and other means, they would encourage the nonwasteful taking of walrus.

To facilitate that process, the Eskimo Walrus Commission also conducted an extensive series of interviews (through its traditional ecological knowledge survey) in the spring of 2004 with four generations of Native hunters from five villages: Diomede, Gambell, Savoonga, Shishmaref, and Wales. With an aim to "enhance the well-being of Pacific walrus as a natural and cultural resource," these conversations captured the views, practices, and perspectives of both elder and younger hunters and found that many in the younger generation now shared the nonwasteful orientation of their elders.[39] While some, such as Asigrook's son, moved out of the area and didn't hunt much, others stayed, worked, and continued the centuries of traditional, subsistence existence.

Native Alaskans depend on their subsistence harvest of Pacific walrus for more than food. Their cultural values, lifestyle, and economy are intertwined with the fate of this funny-looking animal to such an extent that the actions of one affect the actions of the other. This interconnectedness is the basis of traditional culture.

Native subsistence hunters have a very deep relationship with the animals they hunt. "It's not just nutrition, it's not just ceremonial, it's not just religious," Gambell hunter Merle Apassingok said. "That's how God made us. God created us. God picked us, handpicked us for this region, this spot right here."[40]

Subsistence hunting still defines these communities. It keeps everyone strong and shapes their interactions. As Shishmaref hunter John Sinnok says, "It bonds us together and that is why we live here in this community. If we didn't want walrus, or *oogruk* [bearded seal], or anything we would live in Anchorage where we could live off of Safeway, Fred Meyers or Wal-Mart. But that is not who we are, we are subsistence hunters."[41]

Yet the definition of subsistence hunting has changed. Consumption of walrus meat has declined over the years, and today many village children have never even tasted it. In addition, subsistence hunting now requires cash because the tools for the hunt have changed—motor boats, gas, and guns cannot be made locally. Now one must combine subsistence hunting and participation in the cash economy to make either one feasible. Working does not provide enough cash to live, and hunting without modern equipment cannot yield enough to survive. As Asigrook says, he has to "make the best of two worlds and put them together in order to survive."[42]

One mechanism that helps communities meld their two worlds is a redefinition of the subsistence hunting law so that it better reflects reality on the ground. Both the Eskimo Walrus Commission, as the representative body of subsistence hunting communities, and FWS had problems with the lack of a clear definition for nonwasteful take. For FWS, it made law enforcement more difficult because the lines of what was and wasn't allowed weren't clear. Agents had to understand the complexity of each situation and use their judgment. Native subsistence hunters worried they would break the letter of the law if they didn't bring back the entire walrus, even if that meant taking parts they knew they wouldn't use. There were a number of reasons hunters might not take some parts of the walrus.

One was that different communities used different parts. As Asigrook explained, "We differ, depending on where you're from. . . . In Barrow they don't eat the liver. We do down here [in Gambell]. And here we rarely save the flippers of the walrus and on the mainland, that is a prime piece."[43]

What was harvested could also depend on the walrus itself, as certain parts were more or less valued depending on the age and gender of the animal. For instance, subsistence hunters treasured the hides of female walrus to make the walrus-skin boats they used for whale hunting because they were smoother, more flexible, and easier to work with than those from older bulls.

The modernization of Native lifestyles further shifted how hunters used walrus parts. It was much easier, for example, to buy a Gore-Tex raincoat that could be repaired than to make one out of walrus intestines. That meant people no longer needed the innards.

Hunting conditions, too, often dictated what could be taken. The weather could change rapidly, and butchering an open carcass on the ice could generate enough heat to thaw the floe. The last thing anybody needed was to suddenly plunge into the sea or be stranded in a storm, meaning that sometimes the most prudent thing to do was to take only the best parts.

The FWS policy on wasteful take didn't reflect these subtleties. Hunters believed it didn't accurately reflect their world, and FWS knew that was true. While everyone agreed that just taking the head or shooting at a walrus in the water without trying to retrieve it were wasteful, for years Native hunters and law enforcement officers had argued over exactly what *did* need to be taken to be legal and constitute subsistence use.

Throughout the 1990s and early 2000s, the Eskimo Walrus Commission lobbied the FWS for a new policy, with Carl Kava, Eskimo Walrus Commission director through 2001, reasoning, "Regulations for wasteful take should be amended to better cater to the local current traditional practices."[44] As a first step, the Eskimo Walrus Commission conducted a "walrus wanton waste survey" from the fall of 1995 until March 1996 that asked hunters what parts they used. The goal was to give FWS the information to alter the policy to make it clearer, more realistic, and more enforceable.[45]

Eight years later, in May 2004, FWS and the Eskimo Walrus Commission jointly issued revised walrus harvest guidelines. The move was significant because the two organizations developed and published them together, and because they recognized the true circumstances in the communities.

The revised guidelines retained the policy Crane had drafted earlier in the 1990s that specified what hunters had to bring back from each walrus harvested: "at a minimum, the heart, liver, flippers, chest skin with attached blubber (coak), some red meat, and the ivory." It also acknowledged for the first time that walrus utilization had changed over time and provided for the validity of different communities using different parts. Significantly, the revised policy installed the measure of allowing hunters to substitute listed parts for others (such as an entire walrus skin instead of the organs and meat of that same walrus), provided they returned "with a *substantial portion* of each walrus harvested."

The joint guidelines also defined the wasteful practices that would trigger a breach of the law. "Failure to return without a substantial portion of each walrus harvested, taking a walrus without immediately making a reasonable effort to retrieve it, or taking a walrus without using a method that ensures its capture and killing are violations." It discouraged hunters from harvesting walrus when they are in the water and noted that "if hunters do so, they should be prepared to recover the walrus immediately after shooting."

The single page of guidelines concealed years of effort and trust-building that had gone into crafting it. The Eskimo Walrus Commission had worked closely with FWS, first to press for change, then to survey hunters on their needs, and last to wordsmith the revised wasteful-take policy. And just as much as the words on the paper, the back-and-forth process signaled an important move toward greater collaboration between the two on law enforcement.

While the policy still needed to define exactly what constituted a "substantial portion," that could wait for another day. The end result represented a remarkable step forward. The new guidelines not only clarified hunting practices by stressing the need to kill what hunters could retrieve, but, for the first time, they let hunters substitute parts. That showed respect for Native hunters' situation and allowed their own definition of subsistence use to enter the equation.

FWS had supported, not undermined, the continuation of the culture by allowing geographic location, circumstances, and cultural traditions to dictate legality of the hunt. At the same time, Native Alaskan involvement in delineating the line between subsistence hunting and poaching intimated they would abide by it and also turn in lawbreakers.

The reporting of headless walrus to FWS is a critical step to reduce headhunting. Villagers commonly know who chopped off walrus heads but are loath to speak up because divulging their names could lead to trouble. As an *Anchorage Daily News* editorial pointed out following the 1996 clashes over the carcasses in Kotzebue Sound, "It's going to take a bigger crackdown among Natives—particularly the elders and hunters of rank—to stem illegal and wasteful kills."[46] They had to take a stand, otherwise their silence implicitly consented to headhunting and would exact a heavy toll on both the walrus and Native society in the future.

Anecdotal evidence shows hunters increasingly have taken to heart the risk poaching poses to the rest of the community. In the spring of 2003, a Native Alaskan hunter reported headless walrus on the ice twenty miles offshore of St. Lawrence Island.[47] FWS mobilized a team and, after flying over tract after tract of the Bering Sea, located the sixteen carcasses. Using traditional law enforcement investigative techniques, six law enforcement agents went to Gambell to interview hunters and other villagers. They knew where the walrus had been killed, so it didn't take long to find out who had hunted there.

"Typically, when a lot of people witness a crime, the bar is raised. The witnesses need to make a choice to either lie to an agent or fess up," Steve Oberholtzer, assistant special agent in charge of FWS in Alaska, later explained.[48]

In conversation after conversation, agents learned how, on May 21,

2003, five men shot 27 walrus from a herd of about 150 animals and took only their tusks.[49] All later pleaded guilty.[50]

Other instances of Native Alaskans reporting headhunting produced similar results. In July 2003, for example, a report from a Native Alaskan provided the impetus for an investigation that ended with FWS charging two hunters from Barrow with shooting and killing six walrus and removing only the heads and tusks. They, too, pleaded guilty.[51]

These cases were successfully prosecuted only through the help of villagers. Without them, nothing could or would have been done. Their involvement and outrage demonstrate a shift in Native attitudes critical to addressing poaching. Because only other hunters see and are affected by walrus headhunting, they are the most effective way to stop it.

The wildlife crime lab's success at identifying wasteful take from carcasses exposed the problem of headhunting and set in motion a series of events—from expanding Operation Whiteout, to the prosecution of poachers and fears of backlash, to a variety of efforts to shift the Native Alaskan mind-set—that heightened awareness and strengthened the willingness to act among the communities.

The situation, however, remains delicate. Walrus are still killed only for their tusks. While many Native Alaskans follow the law and seek help from FWS to stop illegal activities, others don't. An anonymous report in the summer of 2007 revealed 79 headless carcasses in a 40-mile stretch between Elim and Unalakleet in Norton Sound (east of Nome), the highest count in over ten years.[52] This time, the tone of FWS's response differed and the agency carefully emphasized that the dead walrus did not necessarily mean anyone broke the law. "We're on a fact-finding mission to discover what caused the death of these animals and whether it's legal," Oberholtzer said during the ensuing investigation.[53] While its inquiries never yielded enough evidence for charges against a specific hunter, experience had taught the agency not to speculate on whether wasteful take had occurred.

Native Alaskans are not alone in their struggle to conserve a threatened species in the face of strong economic inducements to poach. Many communities around the world have experienced similar challenges and some have met them head-on by creating economically viable alternatives that provide an incentive for conservation. Because they now benefit financially from tourism and hunting revenue, farmers living in east and southern Africa near game reserves and parks have gone from seeing elephants as nuisances that raided crops to viewing them as animals they want to protect. Programs like Zimbabwe's Communal Areas Management Programme for Indigenous Resources (CAMPFIRE) and others like it in Botswana and Namibia have generated significant money for surrounding communities. As a result of these local conservation programs in conjunction with a commercial trade prohibition and public education campaign, elephant numbers have rebounded. So much so that in southern Africa in 1997 and again in 2007 CITES authorized one-off sales of seized ivory from Botswana, Namibia, South Africa (only in 2007), and Zimbabwe (with the latest to be followed by a nine-year resting period of no ivory sales) to buyers found to have adequate domestic controls. Alaskan communities could follow this model of generating revenue from the species' conservation.

The economic reality faced by Native hunters requires change. For subsistence hunting to continue, the public must be assured that limited catches do not hurt the overall population. The last estimate of the size of the Pacific walrus population was conducted in 1990 when researchers calculated it stood at about 200,000 animals. However, the validity of that figure is uncertain because teams surveyed a fraction of the animal's habitat, estimated the numbers in large herds, and could not account for animals in the water. FWS biologists, working in concert with their Russian counterparts (since Pacific walrus habitat is shared between the two areas), improved the methodology and in 2006 conducted a new walrus census using high-altitude thermal infrared scanning.[54] When the 2006 survey results are available in mid-2009, FWS and walrus-hunting communities can use the population estimate in conjunction with other information on behavior and mortality to manage the species and set sustainable harvest levels.

Diversifying the economy makes sense given that walrus are threatened by far more than illegal hunting. Because they are an ice-dependent species, climate change imperils their future survival. At the same time, proposed oil development in the Bering and Chukchi Seas poses an additional hazard to their habitat.[55] Walrus poaching must be addressed within a broader context of these other threats.

The fate of the Inuit and Yu'pik cultures is tied to the fate of the walrus. As Diomede hunter Charles Menadelook said, "We are not going to need walrus to survive, but we are going to need it as a people."[56] As with the whale, the walrus represents a sign of constancy to remind "everybody from toddler to ancient elder that 'We're still here, we know who we are and we will survive no matter what.'"[57] Sustaining the walrus while preserving the integrity of Native families and communities requires the merging of the best of traditional and modern ways of life. As Native communities melt more and more into the new lifestyle, it may mean that one day they won't hunt anymore. But as Asigrook said, "We're just not quite ready for that yet."[58]

Still, as Crane observed on his return trip in 2005 after thirty years of enforcing walrus-hunting regulations in the region, "the change is incredible and progress is being made."[59] The lab's involvement brought focus and understanding to the issue, and helped to grow a shared mission of wildlife law enforcement. While poaching of walrus has not stopped entirely, the lab's work fostered compliance and renewed respect for the walrus and its importance to Native communities and the Alaskan wilderness.

CHAPTER FOUR

Busted for Bear Galls

The traditional Chinese medicine practitioner slashed the shriveled thumb-sized "fig"—a dried bear gallbladder—with a sharp razor. The gallbladder's light weight felt like that of a piece of wood and always surprised her. Gallbladders are pear-shaped sacs that store and concentrate bile, a fluid secreted by the liver to help the body process fatty foods and cholesterol. When food enters the digestive tract, the gallbladder releases bile into the duodenum (the upper part of the small intestine), where it emulsifies fats.[1]

In one hand, she cupped the thin, leathery membrane that encased the dark brown bile that had hardened and crystallized inside through a slow dehydration process. She emptied the odorless chunks of brown crystals from the organ like a package of coarse unrefined cane sugar and then scraped what remained of the precious medicine, worth far more than gold, into her small pile. Because of its high cost, the practitioner used bear bile only in the severest cases and when everything else had failed.

For over three thousand years, bear bile has been seen by the Asian community as one of the best "cold" medicines to "cool the heat" of an illness. In Western parlance, it has anti-inflammatory, antimicrobial, and fever-reducing properties.[2] In fact, it has proven so effective that modern Western medicine uses the chemically synthesized form of the major bear bile acid (ursodeoxycholic acid) to dissolve gallstones and treat cancers, liver cirrhosis, and other diseases. Producing synthetic bear bile has now become a multimillion-dollar industry.[3] As of the early 2000s, China, Japan, and South Korea consumed about 220,400 pounds (110 tons, or 100,000 kilograms) of synthetic ursodeoxycholic acid, with world consumption perhaps double that figure.[4]

Bear bile was a small part of a vast array of potential treatments used in traditional Chinese medicine (also known as TCM, or traditional Asian medicine). TCM employs both hands-on techniques, such as acupuncture, and natural medications to treat pain and illness. It is thousands of years old, and in China and Vietnam the traditional medical systems are officially recognized by their governments as being on a par with Western medicine.[5]

The basic tenets of traditional Chinese medicine were laid out in what is purportedly the oldest medical text in existence, the *Nei Ching*. Legend has it that the *Nei Ching* was compiled by China's "Yellow Emperor" Huang-ti around 2,600 BC and passed down orally until it was recorded in writing in the third century AD.[6] Several medical texts followed, including the *Divine Husbandman's Classic of the Materia Medica* during the Han dynasty (206 BC to AD 220), *Shen Nung Materia Medica* a thousand years later, and pharmacologist Li Shih-chen's 1597 *Compendium of Materia Medica,* all of which detailed the medicinal uses of botanical, mineral, and zoological substances, such as bear bile.[7]

The vast majority of medicines in the Chinese pharmacopeia are made from plants or minerals. Of 12,800 recorded Chinese medications, only a small proportion, about 12 percent, use animal products.[8] While about 1,000 plant and just 36 animal species are used in traditional Chinese medicine, many of the animal parts employed, such as tiger bone, deer musk, and rhino horn, come from threatened or endangered species. Despite their rarity, they are still considered vital because, according to Asian philosophy, one could gain an animal's unique characteristics by ingesting it.

Traditional Asian medicine differs from Western medicine in its emphasis on prevention over cures and its view of the human body as an organic whole. As the *Nei Ching* observed, "To cure disease is like

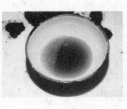

Bear bile.
*(Courtesy of Animals
Asia Foundation)*

waiting until one is thirsty before digging a well."[9] Rather than rely on the strength of the drug for an immediate cure, Oriental medicine heals the illness gradually through treatments that strengthen the patient's own immunity. When someone is sick, instead of concentrating solely on the affected part, as Western medicine does, traditional Chinese medicine practitioners concentrate on helping the patient's body restore its "balance" so that it can fight the disease itself.

This practitioner was going to do just that. She transferred the crystals to a small bowl and reached for her favorite pestle. The cold, gray-green marble implement fit perfectly in her hand, so much so that it almost became an extension of her body. Pressing down with her palm, she moved it in small, circular strokes around the bowl. Not too hard, not too light. While she could buy bear bile as manufactured bile medicines or farmed bile powder, she preferred intact bear gallbladders (which were sold either fresh, frozen, semi-dried, or completely desiccated) so that she could prepare the medicine herself.

Depending on the medical problem at hand, she prepared the bile contained in bear gallbladders differently—sometimes as an ointment or tincture to apply topically, other times in crystal, pill, or powder form to take internally. Each formulation treated a separate ailment, such as hepatitis, jaundice and other liver complaints, high blood pressure, fevers, swelling, gastric or muscle pain, and even eye inflammations such as conjunctivitis.

She mashed the dried bile crystals by rotating the pestle from the inside out. Then she switched, going from the outside in. While others in this modern era used blenders or food processors, she preferred the old-fashioned way so that she could "feel" the consistency of the raw material and avoid possibly destroying its medicinal properties.

She crushed the ever-shrinking crystals until, ten minutes later, pepperlike granules filled the bowl. With tweezers, she pinched a small amount and put it into a gel capsule. When she had filled enough, she put the pills into a container, ready for her patient.

The bear gallbladder used by the practitioner might have come from any one of a number of possible sources. The preferred source of bile has always been the Asiatic black bear (*Ursus thibetanus*). These bears are similar in appearance to the North American black bear except their fur is longer, softer, and shaggier and they weigh a bit less. They also sport a cream-colored crescent-shaped blaze on their chest that gives rise to their common name, moon bear. Asiatic black bears range throughout the forested areas of Asia, including Afghanistan, Pakistan, northern India, Myanmar, southern China, Korea, and Japan. However, high demand for their gallbladders has decimated their populations and today only an estimated 25,000 remain in the wild.[10]

Asia's other bear species have also suffered by virtue of their proximity to the demand for gallbladders. The Malayan sun bear (*Helarctos malayanus*) of Malaysia, Myanmar, Thailand, Vietnam, northern India, and possibly southern China; the sloth bear (*Melursus ursinus*) that lives in the grasslands and forests of India, Sri Lanka, and Nepal; and certain populations (from China, Mongolia, and Bhutan) of the brown bear (*Ursus arctos*) that ranges from Eurasia to North America are all listed in CITES Appendix I (which prohibits commercial trade of the live or dead animals and their parts or derivatives) because of the threat posed by traditional Asian medicine markets. The last of Asia's five bear species, the giant panda (*Ailuropoda melanoleuca*) from China's Sichuan Province, which has fewer than 1,000 animals left, is also threatened and listed in CITES Appendix I, but because of habitat loss rather than the gallbladder trade.

With Asian bear species so rare, countries have looked to alternative sources for bear bile for their traditional medicine. In the 1950s, the Japanese developed a method to synthesize the active ingredient in bear bile, ursodeoxycholic acid (UDC or UDCA). In the early 1980s, North Koreans started "milking" bile from live bears. The Chinese quickly adopted the practice and, according to the CITES Management Authority of China and the Ministry of Forestry, by 1992 they had established 601 farms with 6,632 captive bears.[11] Nevertheless, many Asian consumers prefer wild sources over farmed ones, and whole gallbladders over processed ones, because they feel this bile is more potent.[12]

With commercial trade prohibited for Asian bears, South America's endangered Andean spectacled bear (*Tremarctos ornatus*), brown bears, and polar bears, consumers seek out organs from the moon bear's closest relative, the North American black bear (*Ursus americanus*). Interestingly, North American black bears have high amounts of UDC, on average 39 percent of the total bile acids compared to 8 percent for Asian bears.[13]

North American black bears are relatively plentiful and live in at least forty-one U.S. states and eleven Canadian provinces and territories.[14] Populations numbered between 735,000 and 941,000 animals in the late 1990s, and were roughly split between the United States (with between 339,000 and 465,000 black bears) and Canada (with between 396,000 and 476,000 animals).[15]

Hunting black bears is legal with a license in much of North America.[16] Over 40,000 black bears are killed legally each year, with roughly half (between 22,000 and 25,000) hunted in the United States and half (20,000 to 26,000) in Canada.[17] An equal number is also possibly killed illegally—without a license, out of season, above the bag limits, in unauthorized locations (like a national park), or using prohibited hunting techniques.

In the 1980s, hunters in North America recognized the high value of bear gallbladders and began targeting bears for their parts. After killing the bear (sometimes legally, sometimes illegally), the hunter slit upward from the animal's waist to the lower part of its rib cage to remove the fresh gallbladder, situated beneath the liver. The dark green liquid bile would stretch the thumb-sized muscular membrane until the sac was the size of a plum, or bigger. The size of fresh bear gallbladders varies from those that are tiny like grapes to those that are larger than a fist.[18] Their color varies, too, and spans an awesome spectrum that runs

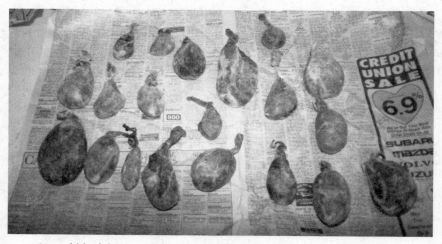

Seized black bear gallbladders. *(Courtesy of Utah Division of Wildlife Resources)*

from yellow to green to brown and many shades and patterns in between.

Careful to avoid spilling any of the bile liquid inside, the hunter ties off what feels like a silicone breast implant with a string and slips the organ into a plastic Ziploc for storage and later sale. While he might also take the bear's leathery, wrinkled forepaws, which are an Asian culinary delicacy reputed to cure male impotence, he'll typically leave the rest of the bear's body to rot. It's an easy way for the hunter to make some extra cash.

Hunters sell the bear gallbladders to local traders, who pass them along to middlemen with contacts in Asian markets. Each person touching the gallbladder and its bile receives a piece of the pie—one that grows the farther away the organ moves from its source. In the early 1990s, a hunter in Idaho received $15 for a bear's gallbladder. The price of that same gallbladder could rocket to $1,500 in Hawaii, with its sizable Asian immigrant market, and up to $55,000 once the powdered bile sold in Korea. Ounce for ounce, bear bile is one of the highest-value commodities on the black market.

Depending on where, when, and how the bear is hunted and where its organs are sold, the transactions might be perfectly legal. U.S. states and Canadian provinces have a patchwork of inconsistent regulations regarding trade in bear gallbladders and other parts that are easy to circumvent. In the United States, in 1999, thirty-five states prohibited the sale of bear gallbladders from bears killed in the state, while five states (Idaho, Maine, Nevada, Vermont, and Wyoming) allowed those sales. Six others (Arkansas, Connecticut, Kansas, Louisiana, North Dakota, and Oklahoma) permitted the trade when the bear was taken legally in another state.[19] Four states—Hawaii, Illinois, Iowa, and Indiana—had no laws governing the sale of black bear parts.[20] While they also had no black bears, the lack of any law allowed bear parts from other jurisdictions to be sold through these states. Canada's provinces had similar inconsistencies.

Given the hodgepodge of regulations and the impossibility of telling if a detached gallbladder originated in a state that permitted its sale and possession, or whether a bear had been lawfully killed, neither hunters nor traders were likely to encounter legal trouble from selling gallbladders.

That is, until wildlife agents across North America focused on the problem.

Rod Olsen, a conservation officer in British Columbia's Conservation Officer Service, the law enforcement arm of the provincial Ministry of Environment, had received during his career a number of complaints from concerned citizens regarding the well-being of the province's 120,000 black bears. British Columbia (B.C.), Canada's westernmost province, was renowned for its rich resources and natural beauty. While bears were plentiful, that abundance didn't mean the population could withstand all threats.

Hunters told Olsen they were having a harder time finding bears, and that when they did, they were usually dead ones with only the paws and gallbladders taken. That type of exploitation worried them, and Olsen, too.

An energetic and outgoing officer in his late twenties, Olsen had joined the service in 1986 after failing to earn his fortune in welding during the early 1980s oil boom in northeastern B.C. and Alberta. With his thick mustache on the blonding side of brown hiding his boyish face, he'd returned to school at the British Columbia Institute of Technology and his longtime love of wildlife, a dream he'd pursued during high school as a seasonal backcountry ranger for B.C. Parks, and became an environment law enforcement officer. He'd spent his first two years with the Conservation Officer Service in Squamish, a remote part of the province, before transferring to the Vancouver area, where he concentrated on pollution investigations. While a regular policeman would've jumped at the chance to be close to the action in the big city, as a wildlife officer Olsen preferred to be nearer the animals he aimed to protect. In 1989, however, his perspective shifted, as he came to appreciate the critical role that urban areas play as a central market and transfer point for trafficking animal parts.

With the hunters' concerns echoing in his head, Olsen received more troubling reports about the province's black bears in 1989. This time, they came from the First Nations people, B.C.'s Native communities. Traders wanted to buy bear gallbladders from the First Nations people to sell in traditional Asian medicine markets in Vancouver and abroad. The province's location on Canada's west coast, close to Asia, together

with its sizable Asian immigrant community and abundant bear populations made it a prime source of gallbladders.

Usually, B.C.'s Native communities took what they needed, about
one or two bears per family each year, primarily for the meat and fat
(which they rendered down into the highly prized West Coast Bannock
Nation bear lard). Provincial law gave the First Nations people unre-
stricted access to bears instead of limiting them to two bears per year as
it did for everyone else. Bear gallbladder dealers wanted to take advantage of that special status to obtain an unlimited supply that could fill
the high domestic and foreign demand.

Like many other Native peoples, the First Nations people valued
bears for their strength, physical prowess, and sacred power. Bears
possess an extremely keen sense of smell, seven times better than a
bloodhound's and perhaps the best of any animal's.[21] They can sense
prey forty miles away and even detect humans more than fourteen
hours after the people have passed an area.[22] While the "smell" part of
a bear's brain is just average-sized, its extra-large nasal mucous mem-
branes, a hundred times that of a human's, and the vomeronasal
organs in the roof of its mouth heighten its sensitivity.[23]

The value of bears goes beyond Native communities and traditional Chinese medicine. Biologists study bears for solutions to a
range of human health problems, from osteoporosis to organ preservation, and to learn the secrets of hibernation for our own long-distance
space travel. Bears are of great interest because they are unaffected by
the ailments a person would suffer from months of not eating, drink-
ing, or moving—dehydration, kidney failure, bone loss, and gallstones. While not "true" hibernators—they can easily waken—during
the long winter months of sleep the fat and the protein from their mus-
cles and organs sustain them. Yet unlike a person's, their bodies don't
suffer, because bears recycle the nitrogen in their urea, a component of
urine produced when tissues break down, to make new protein and
restore their tissues. If they didn't, it would build up as it does for people and become toxic.[24]

For centuries, British Columbia's First Nations people hunted bears
and used them in a variety of cultural contexts, including ceremonies
and for body paints, cosmetics, food, clothing, and blankets. They had
a long-standing tradition of reverence for bears; when they killed and

used the animals, they employed humane hunting practices and wasted as little of the animal as possible.

The Native leaders had concerns about the traders' proposition that they kill, and waste, more than they could use all in the name of profit—and so did Olsen. Given hunters' reports of harder-to-find bears and intact carcasses missing only their gallbladders and paws, Olsen suspected that bears were being killed solely for their valuable parts rather than as trophies or for meat. Like law-abiding hunters and the Native leaders, Olsen hated the waste. He supported hunting; it was a way of life in northwestern Canada, but the unregulated killing of animals for profit was not. While not illegal, squandering the resource crossed an ethical boundary that condemned misuse.

Olsen figured the killing for bear parts was probably significant if the First Nations were seeking government help. Like Alaska's Native communities, First Nations people not only had different wildlife harvest rights but also tended to solve problems internally. The concern had likely become too large for them to handle alone. Plus, the First Nations' apprehensions coincided with hunters' anecdotal evidence of more wasted bears and fewer live ones in the hinterlands.

Before Olsen could take action to protect the bears, he first needed to know more: What spurred the demand for bear parts and how did they fit into the traditional Asian medicine system? Were the province's bears being killed primarily for their gallbladders? If so, just how high was demand? And would this threaten the future sustainability of the population?

Over the next year, Olsen would try to answer those questions through research and by establishing contacts within the Asian community with the help of his subordinate and fellow conservation officer Ralph Krenz.

While Krenz had darker hair, a more wiry build, and, at six feet, was taller than his boss, he was close in age and intensity to Olsen. Ever since he was thirteen years old, when a conservation officer did a license check on him and his dad while they were fishing in northern Alberta, Krenz had known what he'd wanted to do: wildlife law enforcement. "Ride-alongs" with conservation officers while in high school motivated him further, and in 1983, he graduated from the two-year technical program in fish and wildlife technology at the Northern Alberta Institute of Technology. He followed that with a degree in criminology from Mount Royal College in 1984 and worked a variety of seasonal and temporary positions before settling in with the B.C. Conservation Officer Service in January of 1989. This would be one of his first major assignments and he'd attack it with vigor.

Over the next year, during 1989 and 1990, Olsen and Krenz explored the bear parts market by visiting traditional Asian medicine shops in Vancouver's Chinatown, the second-largest Chinatown in North America after San Francisco. Though called Chinatown, in truth it comprised a diverse community of Chinese, Japanese, Vietnamese, Cambodian, and Korean immigrants. Of the metropolitan area's 2.1 million inhabitants in 2006, there were 400,000 (or 19 percent) ethnic Chinese, 46,000 Korean (2 percent), 30,000 Japanese (1.4 percent), 26,000 Vietnamese (1.25 percent), and 1,500 Cambodian (less than 0.1 percent).[25]

The apothecaries visited by Olsen and Krenz were like old-fashioned candy stores, spotlessly clean with a long counter on one side that served as a central hub where pharmacists dispensed medicines and assisted patients, and walls of shelves filled with transparent glass jars.

These Canadian shops represented just a portion of the market for traditional Chinese medicines worldwide. With over three billion potential consumers in Asia and a billion in China alone,[26] the global market for traditional medicines is worth about $60 billion.[27] The United States makes up a large part of that, and in 2000 roughly 160 million Americans spent about $17 billion on these remedies.[28] The traditional Chinese medicine market is exploding in the Western world due to a variety of factors including enhanced exposure from the Internet, globalization and migration of Asians to Western countries, and increased confidence in the ability of traditional Chinese medicine and practices to manage pain, especially that associated with chronic conditions and incurable (with Western medicine), debilitating diseases. Today, a significant proportion of the population in North America and Europe— 42 percent in the United States, 70 percent in Canada, 75 percent in France, 48 percent in Australia, and 38 percent in Belgium—have tried alternative medicines and practices at least once.[29]

Throughout the 1990s and early 2000s, bear parts could be readily found in the United States and Canada. In 2001, a World Society for the Protection of Animals probe surveyed traditional Chinese medicine

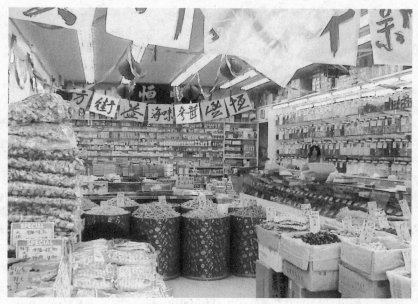

Traditional Asian medicine apothecary shop in Vancouver, Canada.
(Courtesy of Laurel A. Neme)

shops in Canada and four U.S. cities (Chicago, New York, San Francisco, and Washington) and found that 91 percent sold bear parts, including whole fresh, frozen, and dried gallbladders and bile products.[30]

Some of the trade was legal and some illegal. Similar to the United States, in Canada it is provincial and not national law that governs the trade. In 1991, bears resided in all but one (Prince Edward Island) of Canada's provinces and territories. Of these, six (British Columbia, Northwest Territories, Saskatchewan, Manitoba, Quebec, and Nova Scotia) allowed the sale of bear parts and five (Yukon, Alberta, Ontario, New Brunswick, and Newfoundland) did not.[31] Yet even where the *sale* of parts was prohibited, their *possession* was often legal. In 1998, for example, Alberta and New Brunswick both allowed the possession of bear gallbladders. That meant an individual could not be charged for owning a large number of bear gallbladders unless an enforcement officer first obtained evidence of a sale.[32]

Olsen recognized the complexity of the legal situation but remained concerned about the potential threat to the sustainability of bear populations from demand for their parts. Had the intact bear carcasses who'd forfeited their organs been killed solely for their high-value parts? If so, was this market significant enough to trigger a drop in Canada's black bear populations to an unsustainable level?

British Columbia's bears faced demand for gallbladders from several sources. An influx of Asian immigrants into Vancouver strengthened local domestic markets for the organ. After Toronto, Vancouver was Canada's second most ethnically diverse city and attracted a constant stream of immigrants. At the same time, that influx linked local animal parts dealers to traditional Chinese medicine markets in Asia and thus extended the market for organs from British Columbia's bears.

In Asia, demand for traditional Chinese medicine was expanding due to the boom of their economies. From the 1960s to 1990s, South Korea, Taiwan, Singapore, and Hong Kong, referred to as the "Asian tigers," abandoned import substitution and replaced it with export promotion policies. Other countries followed suit, and during a twenty-five-year period from 1965 to 1990, the four "tigers" plus Japan, Indonesia, Malaysia, and Thailand experienced extraordinary and sustained economic growth, an event often referred to as the East Asian Miracle. The affluence of Asian economies resulted in the increased wealth of their citizens and intensified demand for previously unaffordable consumer goods, including animal parts. Simultaneously, the direct linkages with Vancouver residents allowed and prompted bear hunters from British Columbia to connect with these ready and lucrative markets.

Yet supplying those markets had the potential to hurt Canada's black bear populations. If just 0.1 percent of the 1.3 billion potential consumers in China, Taiwan, Japan, South Korea, and North Korea in 1991 each bought a single bear gallbladder, North America's entire black bear population could be wiped out.

British Columbia might bear the brunt of that threat. The province's southern and eastern neighbors, Washington State in the United States and Alberta in Canada, had recently (in 1989) imposed new prohibitions on trade in bear gallbladders. This meant that British Columbia, where it was legal to buy and sell the organs, would become a safe haven for dealers. It would be a simple matter to transport bear parts across jurisdictions and claim that they came from British Columbia. Consequently, the province faced a dual menace: hunters would seek out its bears to meet demand and traffickers would use its looser laws to "launder" the gallbladders of bears killed elsewhere.

Canada kept minimal records on the bear parts trade. No province (except Nova Scotia) required reports for bear parts leaving their jurisdiction.[33] At the same time, exports were growing. Traffic at the Port of Vancouver, the largest in Canada, was growing steadily. Container traffic swelled from 1.1 million tons (1 million metric tonnes) in 1982 to over 13.2 million tons (12 million metric tonnes) in 2002, an average annual growth rate of more than 13 percent.[34] While Customs agents looked out for potential hazards that might be entering the country, they didn't watch what was going out. Parts from Canada's bears could be slipping across the sea with nobody the wiser.

Anecdotal information from hunters of it being harder to find bears in the wild areas outside Vancouver along with contacts among dealers and the Asian community led Olsen to believe that harvests of North American black bears were on the rise due to growing demand from traditional Chinese medicine markets in Vancouver and overseas.

But he had no way of knowing for sure.

To address that lack of knowledge, he proposed launching an investigation into the bear gallbladder trade. At first he suggested a plainclothes investigation into stores that might be selling the organs, and later revised his proposal to an undercover operation into the dealers.

While no law forbade trading bear parts specifically, Olsen proposed using the provincial Wildlife Act, which prohibited all wild-meat trafficking, by arguing that bear gallbladders were consumed and thus constituted wild meat.

Because his agency, the B.C. Conservation Officer Service, didn't want to pursue the cost and risk of an investigation if it had no chance of success, Olsen went to the province's Crown Counsel, or prosecutor, Alan Blair, to assess the likelihood of convictions for the undercover investigation. Blair agreed the proposed investigation could succeed legally. However, at that time the Wildlife Branch, also in B.C.'s Ministry of Environment, decided to alter the wild-meat trafficking regulation to allow buying and selling of bear gallbladders. Fur traders had been pressuring the agency to change the law, and the agency's own wildlife biologists said the province's healthy bear populations warranted legalization of the trade. As a result, the Conservation Officer Service postponed Olsen's proposed covert investigation so that Olsen could take advantage of the paper trail that the new regulation would generate.

In late 1989, the Ministry of Environment amended the Commercial Activities Regulation of B.C.'s Wildlife Act (B.C. Reg. 338/82) to allow licensed fur traders to buy and sell bear gallbladders legally.

Throughout Canada, black bears are classified as a game animal that can be hunted with an appropriate license. Within the game animal designation, British Columbia categorized black bears as a "furbearing" species. That label authorized fur traders to purchase and sell their pelts. It also authorized trappers (who purchased the rights to hunt animals within a registered area on private land or a trapline) to kill the animals (in addition to regular hunters), and one person might be both a fur trader and a hunter and/or trapper.

The provincial government required separate licenses for hunters, trappers, and fur traders. Each license gave the licensee a unique number and specified particular rules, quotas, and practices. The government required fur traders to report on all merchandise they accepted or bought from hunters or trappers. These reports had to include the name of the hunter or trapper who supplied the item and his or her license number. That way, the government ensured that the royalty (tax) was paid on the pelts and also verified that the hide came from a legally harvested animal.

Legalizing the sale of bear gallbladders would expand the list of acceptable products for fur traders to buy and sell and require them to submit detailed records on their purchases. The change in the law meant that in order to trade bear gallbladders, all one had to do was apply for a fur trader's license, pay the nominal fee, and submit monthly reports.

While Olsen had lost the initial fight to investigate the bear gallbladder trade, the delay ultimately provided stronger ammunition that he would need to challenge it. The change in the law, while legalizing the trade, would establish records on buyers, sellers, and volumes of sales that would make it easier for Olsen to go after the culprits who circumvented it.

In the spring of 1990, after the new regulations allowing trade in bear gallbladders were in place, Olsen and Krenz went through the reports from the hunting season. As a requirement of their license, fur traders promised to complete monthly reports disclosing all of their purchases, including bear parts. The reports were supposed to provide the name and license number of the hunter or trapper who sold the items to the fur trader.

But the accounts didn't add up.

While the hunting and trapping licenses had unique numbers that applied to a single organ, the gallbladders themselves had no distinct identification. Unlike other animal parts, such as rams' horns, which could be tattooed or otherwise individually identified, permanently marking bear gallbladders was impossible. Fur traders capitalized on this inability and concealed the actual number of gallbladders they were circulating by reusing a single valid hunter or trapper license, good for one organ, for multiple organs. They simply claimed that the legitimate hunter or trapper license number, received for an organ bought earlier, applied to whatever gallbladder they had on hand. Because there was no way to match the license number to a specific gallbladder, they could carry out this ruse indefinitely.

Olsen and Krenz reviewed the fur traders' reports and saw a pattern of license numbers. Comparing the sellers' numbers in a spreadsheet, they found that one bear-hunting license was typically used for five gallbladders, and those were only the ones the trader reported. Using information from the officers' regular intelligence contacts, including hunters who lawfully sold bear gallbladders to traders, Olsen and Krenz knew that fur traders frequently failed to declare many other organs. Fur traders often underreported their inventory to minimize the royalties (taxes) paid to the provincial government. They also kept numbers low so as not to arouse unwanted attention from the government, which might decide trade was too large and take actions to limit it.

To address the deceit, Olsen proposed opening what would be the agency's first undercover investigation into bear trafficking, called Operation Ice Bear, with an up-and-coming fur trader, Sang Ho Kim, as the initial target. Olsen knew from hunters and trappers who sold their bear gallbladders to Kim that the dealer was not reporting all of his purchases. He also knew Kim had knowledge of the law. The trader had received official letters about what was required of him and had stated to uniformed officers when he'd filed his reports that they were complete.

Certain that Kim had bought and sold undeclared bear galls, Olsen planned to have an undercover officer sell Kim bear gallbladders. Then, when Kim failed to report the purchase, Olsen would have proof of his cheating.

Olsen decided to take advantage of Kim's position as a relative newcomer to the trade. As such, the dealer had struggled to convince the tight-knit circles of buyers in Asia that he offered the real product. Fake bear gallbladders were as common as knockoff designer handbags because distinguishing the gallbladder's origin from the organ alone was difficult. Gallbladders from bears and pigs appear remarkably similar, although experts assert their odors differ and that bear gallbladders retain a slight honey smell. To establish the organs' authenticity and his reliability as a seller, Kim sought out intact bears so that he could remove the organs in front of his clients. He'd asked several Vancouver-based taxidermists for the whole animal and one of them, offended by the wastefulness, complained to Olsen. Olsen seized the opportunity and advised the taxidermist to give Kim the name of a supplier, Mike Sinnott. In reality, however, Sinnott was Mike Girard, a conservation officer in Powell River who would pose as a cash-strapped "falling" or logging contractor working British Columbia's coast and looking to make some money from gallbladders on the side.

To prepare for Kim and Girard's meeting, Olsen and Krenz put out a province-wide request for bear gallbladders. While Kim wanted intact bears to establish himself as a reliable seller, he primarily wanted the organs, which were small, easy to smuggle, and easy to sell. The conservation officers had promised themselves not to hurt any bears in their investigation and to use only parts from already dead bears or those killed for another reason. But finding those animals wasn't easy. Eventually, a garbage-habituated bear foraging at a dump that had been relocated several times had to be killed.[35] Olsen would use this animal's parts for the investigation. That, in turn, might help save hundreds of other bears.

Because neither of the two agents knew how to prepare a bear's gallbladder, they experimented on the one from this sow. Traffickers recognize their product readily, so if Olsen and Krenz got it wrong, Kim would quickly "make" Girard as a fraud. Olsen tied off the gallbladder with string and hung it up with heat and a fan to dry. A few days later, the two officers checked their handiwork. The bladder had collapsed into a flattened chunk. Worse, it was as hard as a rock. Olsen cut into it with a penknife but only managed to flake off a few chips. A stronger hunting knife still couldn't dent it and a hammer only shattered it. Despite this evident failure, they continued to test other methods until finally they had a passable supply.

On May 27, 1991, Mike Girard took six gallbladders from the freezer, laid them on the bottom of a white Styrofoam cooler, added ice, and grabbed two dried gallbladders provided by Olsen and Krenz. He slid behind the wheel of his wife's car, a light blue 1978 Firebird. It fit the swagger of his undercover persona far more than his own pickup truck. In his early forties, Girard was older than Olsen and Krenz, and more experienced. He joined British Columbia's provincial park service in 1971 after graduating high school, and continued to work for them full-time after college. A stickler for rules and regulations, he had frequently found himself frustrated with the B.C. Parks' soft approach to wildlife law enforcement. After fourteen years, in 1985, he left to join the conservation service as a "bush cop" patrolling the wild areas to enforce hunting and other wildlife regulations.

He tugged his baseball cap lower and shifted into his role of cash-strapped logger. The false persona wasn't much of a stretch. Girard had spent his early years in remote industrial camps running chain saws and bucking trees in the bush. He headed toward the Coach House Inn on Vancouver's north shore where he'd arranged a meeting with Kim.

When Kim arrived, Girard pulled out the cooler. Kim reached for the first dried gall, raised it to his face, and inhaled slowly. Like the bear it came from, he could tell a lot with his nose. He scratched the gallbladder with a penknife and sniffed again. A sweet honey smell would confirm that the organ was from a bear and not some other animal.

He repeated the process for the rest of the galls. Finally, Kim made an offer: a thousand dollars (Canadian) for everything.[36]

Girard countered with fifteen hundred (Canadian) and, after a little back-and-forth, they agreed on an amount in between: twelve hundred (Canadian) (US$875).

Kim handed over a roll of bills and Girard counted it.

You're a couple hundred short, the undercover officer said.

Acknowledging the error, Kim promised he'd bring the rest of the money next time.

• • •

Over the next two months, in the summer of 1991, Girard staged three undercover meets with Kim, as well as some additional meetings to pick up money. During that time, Girard sold Kim fourteen gallbladders and twenty paws. These contacts let him gain Kim's trust and obtain the evidence he needed to make a strong case against the dealer. This was the first time anybody in the province had obtained firsthand information about the bear gallbladder trade. Because of that, the officers could prove the dealer failed to record all his purchases on his fur trader's reports, and that would allow the agents to establish the illegality of Kim's operation.

Girard cultivated a friendship with Kim and tried to put him, a somewhat nervous man, at ease by taking him on a relaxed cruise down the Fraser River on his disguised government-issue patrol boat. As Kim felt more comfortable, he asked Girard for whole bears—just as he had with the taxidermist. While he'd made the same request several times before and Girard had always responded positively, it had never gone further than talk. Girard figured it was because Kim was reluctant to fully commit to wildlife trafficking. Yet this time the two made concrete plans.

Kim intended to bring his South Korean buyers to British Columbia and cut out the gallbladders in front them. Because the dealer didn't have a way to store a bear carcass (and given the summer heat, it'd go bad quickly), for an extra few hundred dollars Girard offered the use of one of his remote logging camps that had large freezers.

Back in Vancouver, Olsen and Krenz were pleased. They had reviewed Kim's most recent fur trader submissions and confirmed that Kim had failed to report all of his bear gallbladder sales, as required by his license. With Girard's undercover sales, they could prove that Kim was cheating. But to demonstrate that this relationship represented more than a few one-off sales, the officers would have to locate Kim's business accounts and extra stock of gallbladders, which he probably kept at his house. To get a search warrant, they needed one final sale. This would allow the agents to follow Kim to his residence with fresh evidence (bear galls) so that they could apply for a search warrant and be able to say beyond a reasonable doubt that the bear galls were at the residence while the application for the warrant was taking place. Sometimes if there is too much of a time delay between when the evidence arrives at a location and the application, the warrant will not be granted, since there is the possibility that the items would have been moved in the time frame and there would be no reasonable grounds to believe that the evidence was there. The search warrant required them to demonstrate probable cause of a legal violation and show reasonable grounds that Kim used this location as a place where he trafficked the gallbladders. The proposed transaction at Girard's logging camp would do the trick nicely.

However, it was not to be. Girard slipped a disk in his back during his regular duties as a conservation officer in remote Powell River. Now he needed surgery and would be out of commission for months.

That meant they'd have to start over and introduce Kim to a new "buyer."

Olsen turned to the most recent hire on his team, B.C. Conservation Officer Dan LeGrandeur, as a replacement. He'd make a final transaction (although it wouldn't be at Girard's logging camp since, ostensibly, the two didn't know each other).

Because of his lack of experience, LeGrandeur opposed the idea. While he'd helped with surveillance and participated in other, nonvisible parts of the operation, he had never gone undercover for a "meet" with a bad guy. However, as the newest agent, he didn't have much choice. Neither Krenz nor Olsen were viable candidates because people in the Asian community would recognize them. Soon, the local taxidermist passed LeGrandeur's name on to Kim and they set up a meeting.

Yet LeGrandeur had a problem. He had little to offer Kim. Because this rendezvous was at the tail end of the operation, the conservation officers had few bear parts left: just one gallbladder and some paws. Olsen tried to boost the junior officer's confidence by promising that Kim would never know the difference if they doctored up pig galls. Over the next several days, the conservation officers carved fat deposits off pig organs and replicated the honey smell by painting bile from an unsalable ruptured bear gall on their exteriors.

The day of the last sale finally arrived. On March 14, 1992, posing as a cowboy from Kamloops, LeGrandeur swung his red Bronco into a McDonald's parking lot less than a half block away from the agents' government office. Olsen and Krenz observed from a nearby car.

LeGrandeur pulled into the spot opposite Kim's white Lumina van and motioned the Asian man into his vehicle. With Kim settled in the front seat, the agent handed over a bag of gallbladders and watched him inspect the first gall. The dealer scratched it with a penknife, sniffed, and angrily pronounced it a fraud.

LeGrandeur stuttered while his mind raced. He'd relied so much on Olsen's confidence that he hadn't rehearsed what to say if Kim uncovered the deception.

Kim took another gallbladder from the bag and declared it a fake from pig.

LeGrandeur recovered quickly. He acted surprised and angry, shouting, "What do you mean they're pig? The buddies I cowboy with asked me to sell 'em. I'm gonna kill those guys. I'm so sorry. I can't believe they screwed me over!"

The performance worked. Kim clucked in empathy.

The dealer scrutinized another and comforted LeGrandeur by noting that this one really *was* from a bear.

Kim examined the rest and offered the agent C$80 for the lot. LeGrandeur was anxious to complete the sale and didn't want to dicker. But he knew that if he accepted the amount outright, Kim would get suspicious. He countered with C$90 (US$65) and Kim agreed.

With the gallbladders sold, the two men turned to the bear paws and laid out twenty on the floor of Kim's van. Satisfied with the haul, Kim offered C$5 (US$3.65) apiece. LeGrandeur agreed and the dealer handed over a wad of cash.

Olsen and Krenz followed Kim to his home, where they watched him carry the cooler they knew contained LeGrandeur's bear parts into his house, and phoned LeGrandeur, who was waiting for the call outside a judge's house. LeGrandeur obtained the warrant and raced to Kim's residence to hand the signed paper to Olsen. The legalities now covered, Olsen and his team searched Kim's residence. There they found not only Kim's records but a whole frozen bear carcass, a cache of paws, and almost one hundred dried gallbladders—a sizable stash.

The probe against Kim led to other dealers, and ultimately, Olsen's Operation Ice Bear involved cases against five unlawful dealers, including Kyu Hak Yon, who was also put on trial. The undercover bear gall trafficking investigation into Kim and others led to several follow-up covert law enforcement operations. These probes focused on other parts of the supply chain, namely the hunters who supplied the organs and the shops that sold them. Agents acted as middlemen who bought gallbladders from the hunters. They also posed as Asian tourists, the purchasers of the final product, and went to shops where bear galls were being sold. The web of bear parts trafficking is so wide and its threat to bears so large that they necessitated an investigation with such a broad scope.

To slow the trade, the agents first needed to prove their case against Kim. They would have to demonstrate that, contrary to the requirements of his fur trader's license, Kim failed to report his bear gallbladder sales. To do so, they would have to verify that Kim's gallbladder stockpile did, in fact, come from bears and not some other animal.

With the evidence in his possession, Olsen called the FWS wildlife forensic laboratory.

Could the lab confirm that the gallbladders came from bear?

CHAPTER FIVE

Bear Bile . . . or Not?

While Olsen investigated Kim in Canada, U.S. agents in Wyoming were investigating a similar case.

In the late 1980s, Wyoming resident Mike Weston* discovered a new business opportunity while watching a CNN news report on the bear parts trade. Bear parts are extremely valuable, the report said. Gallbladders are worth between $1,000 and $5,000 each.

Weston figured that was easy money. He could buy the organs cheaply, and even if he sold them for a lot less than what the report said, still make big bucks.

What was the downside?

Regulations vary, the CNN report continued, as if in response to the unasked question. In some states, like California, selling bear galls is prohibited, while in other states, like Idaho, it's fine.

Weston reckoned it wouldn't be hard to avoid problems. Hunting bear in most U.S. states and Canadian provinces was okay with a license, so all he'd have to do was sell the parts in a place where it was legal.

In July 1990, Weston offered 160 frozen bear gallbladders to a buyer on the phone for $150 each. It was a fair price but he was willing to dicker a bit. He'd bought them last spring from a dealer in Wyoming for $20 apiece, so he stood to make a bundle no matter what.

On the other end of the phone, FWS special agent Bill Harrison† hes-

---

*Not his actual name.
†Not his actual name.

itated. Based in Nevada, Harrison had been working undercover for most of the year, posing as a buyer of bear parts to build his credibility among animal parts dealers throughout the western United States. Weston was his latest contact. Harrison needed to know where Weston had bought the gallbladders, and persuading him to supply the information was crucial. No federal prohibition existed and every state and province had different laws regarding bear parts sales, so Weston's answer would determine if the transaction was legal or not. At that time, eight states—Idaho, Maine, New Hampshire, New York, Vermont, Virginia, West Virginia, and Wyoming—authorized the commercial sale of gallbladders and twenty-eight states with bear populations banned it. However, some of these, like Connecticut, allowed it when the bears were legally killed in another state.[1] Knowing the location and legality of the hunt *and* the location and legality of the sale were critical to making a case against Weston.

Over the next five weeks, Harrison and Weston talked a dozen times, with the agent pressing for information about the origin of the gallbladders and the legality of the sale. Weston told the undercover agent he'd collected the bear galls from ten outfitters in Colorado, Idaho, and Wyoming.

While many bear parts enter the trade legally, the high value of bear gallbladders spurs poaching. A four- or five-ounce gallbladder is far easier to carry than a two-hundred-pound bear hide or a nine-foot trophy, and, on a per-pound basis, more lucrative, too.

Just as officers in Canada had, over the past decade FWS agents had noticed increased illegal hunting of bears and proliferation of their gallbladders in the market. In the 1980s, several major investigations into illegal bear parts trafficking uncovered the breadth of the poaching spurred by the trade in bear parts. Operation Berkshire, a two-and-a-half-year investigation ending in 1989, resulted in Massachusetts and New York State environmental agencies charging seven men with 300 counts of hunting violations. In the late 1980s, a three-year federal FWS probe code-named Operation Smoky in the Great Smoky Mountains identified almost 370 illegal bear kills, seized 300 bear gallbladders, and made arrests in Tennessee, Georgia, and North Carolina. Similarly, the four-year Operation Trophy Kill led to the arrests of over 50 people in 12 states across the country for poaching of bears and other species.[2]

More recently, the National Park Service, FWS, and the Virginia

Department of Game and Inland Fisheries jointly undertook a three-year undercover sting into bear poaching in the Shenandoah National Park region, called Operation SOUP (for Special Operation to Uncover Poaching),[3] that ended in 1999. Operation SOUP triggered the arrest of over two dozen people for more than fifty wildlife violations related to bear poaching and illegal trade in bear parts.

A host of additional cases focused not on poaching but on the sale of gallbladders in traditional Chinese medicine markets, with most states that have either bears or an Asian population engaged in the trade. In California, a three-year investigation in 1988 resulted in the arrests of 51 Asian traders. In 1991, Alaska officers halted two trafficking operations, one with 173 bear galls purchased in Quebec and another with 385 pounds of frozen bear galls and paws from Idaho. In Colorado's first major bear parts trafficking investigation in 1992, Operation Betelgeuse, agents arrested nine people. Virginia state game agency's Operation VIPER, a follow-up probe to the antipoaching Operation SOUP that ended in 2004, targeted consumers (versus suppliers as did Operation SOUP) of bear parts and documented nearly 500 state violations and more than 200 federal violations by over 100 people in seven states and the District of Columbia.

The specific number of gallbladders involved in the trade is unknown because much is illegal and thus unreported. Yet each dealer typically traffics hundreds of gallbladders. For example, the 1994 arrest of a Los Angeles–based entrepreneur caught the dealer with 164 illicit bear galls, but he'd previously boasted to undercover agents of his capacity to handle large orders of 400 or more.[4]

While these investigations show how widespread the trade is, its full extent is difficult to determine. In a 1996 Humane Society of the United States report on the trade, an FWS agent projected that "for every poaching case uncovered at least one hundred go undiscovered."[5] Other estimates are more conservative and vary from a one-to-one ratio of legal to illegal bear kills to two or three bears taken illegally for every ten legal ones.[6]

The market is pervasive. In 2000, the World Society for the Protection of Animals investigated sixty-five traditional Chinese medicine shops in seven North American cities (New York, San Francisco, Chicago, and Washington, D.C., in the United States and Toronto, Montreal, and Vancouver in Canada) and found that 78 percent sold

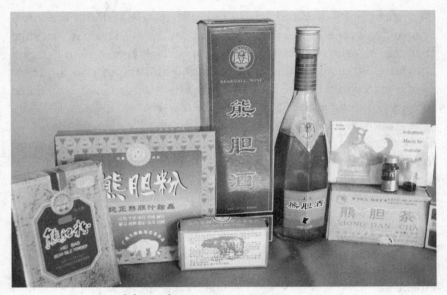

Bear bile products. *(Courtesy of Animals Asia Foundation)*

bear gallbladders or bile products.[7] Weston's case symbolized yet one more opportunist capitalizing on this profitable market.

On September 7, 1990, Harrison and Weston met at a suburban Denver motel to finalize their deal. From Harrison's perspective, the Colorado location was perfect because it meant the transaction would take place in a state that prohibited the trade. After haggling over price, the two agreed on $24,000 for a lot of purportedly 188 bear gallbladders.

Weston offered the agent twelve clear plastic bags with numbers scrawled on the outsides in black Sharpie. Presumably, each contained the number of gallbladders indicted, but there was no way to confirm it. The squashed organs had frozen together and the agent couldn't tell where one ended and another began.

Harrison handed Weston a wad of forty $100 bills and said the remainder, $20,000, was in his car. As the agent turned toward his vehicle to retrieve the cash, he stretched and placed his hands behind his neck, a signal to his surveillance team. Seconds later, federal agents stormed the men and arrested Weston.

•   •   •

A few days later, Special Agent Harrison put down his pen and reread the complaint against Weston that he'd just signed. The U.S. attorney in Denver would charge Weston with violating the Lacey Act, a federal law prohibiting interstate shipment of wildlife taken or possessed illegally. By going from Wyoming to Colorado, Weston had crossed state lines to transact a sale that violated an underlying state law.

By Weston's calculation, and those of other traders as well, the risks if caught were minimal compared to the potential rewards. Usually, the charges were only minor state misdemeanors with negligible penalties. And the dealer could always defend himself by claiming the contraband came from pigs, which was legal. That's exactly what Weston did.

But Special Agent Harrison had what seemed to be incontrovertible evidence: the 188 gallbladders Weston had sold him. All the prosecutor needed for a conviction was proof the gallbladders came from bear.

The large volume of organs was especially useful because of its considerable commercial value, worth well over the Lacey Act's recommended $350 "floor"; that justified a more serious felony charge and had tougher penalties. Federal sentencing guidelines based the punishment on the market value of the animal or animal product involved in the crime. The higher its value, the stiffer the sentence. When Harrison confirmed that the organs were, in fact, bear gallbladders, he'd have a solid case that would act as a deterrent to other dealers. Without that verification, however, he'd have no case.

The agent turned to the one place that could give him what he needed: the wildlife forensics lab.

In September 1990, Harrison reached Ed Espinoza, the top chemist at the FWS wildlife forensics laboratory, at a San Francisco convention after days of tracking him down. With little preamble, he explained what he wanted: authentication of Weston's bear gallbladders.

Standing at the crowded bank of telephones, Espinoza told Harrison to send the evidence to the lab and that he'd work on it when he got back. But when they'd hung up, the reality of the problem hit the scientist. How could he tell if a gallbladder came from bear when he had only the lone organ?

What made a bear a bear? The vast majority of the lab's work focused on finding out what kind of animal a piece of evidence came from. If it was from a protected species, the act of selling its parts was usually a crime. While the North American black bear had no such designation, and thus had no overarching legal protection, laws and regulations in certain states and provinces prohibited traders from selling their gallbladders. Proving that the gallbladders Weston had sold were from bears was necessary because it wasn't criminal to sell gallbladders from other species.

While the question of what makes a bear a bear seems simple, the task of identifying the unique characteristics of a species based on only a single part is not. If these gallbladders had had a bit of liver attached, it would have been possible to do a DNA test that would have told the scientists definitively if they were bear. But the acidity of the bile acids is harsh and corrosive to proteins and DNA alike. They had to find another way.

Sometimes there is little to differentiate a body part from one species or another. For tusks of mammoths and modern elephants, five months of experiments revealed a measurable difference between the angle of the fine, curved lines radiating from the center of the tusk, called Schreger lines.

For each part of each species, the characteristic may differ. With shahtoosh shawls woven from the fine, dense underfur of the rare Tibetan antelope (*Panthelops hodgsonii*), microscopic comparisons between it and wool from legally obtainable cashmere goats revealed no difference. However, in the mid-1990s, the lab's mammalogist and hair identification expert, Bonnie Yates, discovered that large, rounded cells completely filled the shafts of the animal's outer guard hairs, like pebbles packed in a tube. In contrast, the smaller diameter guard hair shaft from cashmere goats appeared solid and dark, nothing like the Tibetan antelope. Because a few stray guard hairs were always mixed in with the underfur in the shawls, that revelation led to the successful prosecution of cases against shahtoosh dealers in the United States, England, and Asia, with Yates testifying at a Hong Kong trial involving over $1 million worth of shahtoosh shawls.

What would the telling characteristic be for bear gallbladders? Did a bear's gallbladder even have an identifying characteristic, something that was unique and not present in any other species? And if it did, could Espinoza find it?

The scientist started as he always did: by reviewing the scientific literature. Whenever possible, he avoided starting an investigation from scratch by first looking to other scientists' work for ideas he could incorporate or adapt. He never confined himself solely to veterinary or forensic journals, and with good reason. During his research, he found inspiration in a human surgical medical journal (*Journal of Surgical Research*), in an article by A. C. MacDonald and C. N. Williams, two researchers seeking nonsurgical treatments for gallstones.

People develop gallstones when their bile is lithogenic, meaning that it forms calculi, or solids, made of mineral salts, which occurs when we fast for long periods. Bears don't. Even when they hibernate and don't eat for months, bears never get gallstones. MacDonald and Williams planned to exploit that fact by uncovering what made a bear's bile different and seeing if they could use that quality to cure gallstones without surgery. "One could anticipate that animals subjected to those risks known to cause bile lithogenicity would either develop gallstones or demonstrate some protective mechanism against such an occurrence, i.e., the production of UDC."[8]

MacDonald and Williams hypothesized that bears produced high levels of the specialized bile salt ursodeoxycholic acid (UDC or UDCA), which in turn protected them from gallstone disease. "Cholesterol gallstones are not reported in Ursidae [bears], probably because of the large bile acid pool and high UDC content," they concluded.[9]

For MacDonald and Williams, the bears' lack of gallstones meant ursodeoxycholic acid might hold the key to an effective and acceptable therapy to dissolve, rather than surgically remove, gallstones.[10] For Espinoza, it told him where to start looking for the species-defining characteristics of a bear's gallbladder: in its bile acids.

Ursodeoxycholic acid occurs naturally in mammalian bile, but usually only in trace amounts.[11] Espinoza reasoned that the key to establishing the identifying characteristic of black bear bile would rest in the *levels* of the acid. But before he could compare acid levels to the bile of other species, he'd have to figure out how to measure the levels.

He turned back to the gallstone study for clues. MacDonald and Williams used thin layer chromatography (TLC), a technique to separate mixtures, in their study. But in their sample of only five bears, they'd found a lot of variation in levels, with higher UDC concentrations in older bears than in younger ones.[12] Because TLC seemed to pick up the slightest variations between individuals of the same species, Espinoza felt it might be too sensitive for his purposes and make it harder to spot significant differences between species.

Espinoza needed both confidence in the levels of bear bile acids and the ability to compare them with other species. Reading the literature and talking with other scientists, he soon learned of Lee Hagey, a graduate student at the University of California–San Diego studying how bile could be used to determine what made one species different from another. Hagey used a process called high performance liquid chromatography (HPLC) to separate out the chemical structures of bile from numerous different species.

Espinoza called Hagey in September 1990 and Hagey explained that because bile was a latecomer to the world of molecular evolution, bile acid differences would help him understand the evolution of vertebrates. Most molecules in the human body are the same as those in any other animal. We have the same chemicals as a bear, for instance, with the same fats, sugars, and amino acids in both species. "It's just that we have them in different proportions and might use them in alternative ways," Hagey noted.[13]

But bile doesn't have the same structural constraints as those chemicals; it doesn't have a billion years of history locking it in place. As evolution occurred, bile took on new patterns, so that bile in bear is different from bile in a kangaroo or in humans.

Espinoza was thrilled to learn about Hagey's techniques and wasted no time in practicing them and then using them on the gallbladders collected by Harrison.

A few days later, Espinoza waited outside the evidence unit while the evidence technician collected the gallbladders he had requested.

Within a few minutes she had plopped a dozen large plastic bags on an empty utility cart. She jotted the date on her forms, verified the evidence tag numbers, noted the transfer from her unit to the scientist, and asked Espinoza to initial the changes. With the chain of custody clearly documented, she wheeled the evidence gallbladders to the door.

Espinoza rolled the cart down the stark, hospital-like hallway to his chemistry lab. Three black horseshoe-shaped counters filled the room while, above them, glass cabinets neatly stocked with solutions, beakers, and other equipment broadcast the chemistry lab's purpose.

Espinoza placed the bags under the biohazard cover to unfreeze overnight and secured the room. The next day, he and his assistant, Jo Ann Shafer, untwisted the ties and revealed a golden brown mass of defrosted gallbladders.

Taking a deep breath, Espinoza stuck his gloved hand in the middle of the slimy mess and wrapped his fingers around the first thing they touched—a squishy, honey-colored organ, about the size and consistency of a boneless chicken breast. He then slipped it onto a waiting glass dish.

Its outward appearance wasn't distinctive. The gallbladder could just as easily have come from a pig as a bear. Their size and shape made them virtually identical. He attached a numbered tag to the organ for future identification and reached in again. Eventually, he separated them into 182 galls in total, not the 188 Harrison believed he'd bought.

Espinoza peeled off his gloves, opened the equipment cabinet, and grabbed what he'd need for the first round of analysis: B-D syringes, 1½-inch-bore needles, glass droppers, vials, caps, and a plastic storage tray. He had decided to analyze each sample with both procedures: the more sensitive TLC and the less sensitive HPLC. In forensic science, findings must conform to certain standards, known as the Daubert (or their predecessor, Kelly Frye) principles. Named after a legal case, these principles maintain that expert scientific opinion, which includes both methodology and results, must be peer reviewed and generally accepted by the relevant scientific community before it can be admissible in court. Because neither the TLC nor HPLC procedures had been adequately vetted for this kind of species identification, Espinoza would use both to act as a cross-check, which in turn would enhance the acceptability of his analysis.

Holding a gallbladder with one gloved hand, he cut into the bile sac with a razor-sharp surgical knife, inserted a needle into the incision, and pulled the plunger until a honey-yellow fluid filled the syringe. Extracting the bile from the middle of the organ instead of its outer layer would ensure that nothing in the external environment could contaminate it.

After removing two milliliters of the liquid, Espinoza transferred the bile from the first evidence gallbladder to a vial. While the organs were potential biohazards that had to be kept under the special hood, the bile itself was innocuous and didn't need the same safeguards. He capped off the vial, labeled it with its own lab evidence number, and put it in the blue plastic tray.

One down, 181 more to go.

Espinoza changed syringes and repeated the procedure. He was used to the monotony of forensic work yet the repetition never lulled his mind. For a chemist, attention to the tiniest details typically meant success or failure.

When he'd finished this first step of bile extraction from the evidence gallbladders, Espinoza set the partially full tray of vials on the counter and duplicated the process a final time with a sample that he knew was from bear. He always did that as a "control" to be certain the method worked.

Now for "step two."

He took a couple of brown jugs of chemical solutions and set them on the counter. Plain white labels announced their contents. The first was MeOH, or methanol, which would flush, or clean, the columns, or tubes, in the machine, to make sure no cross-contamination occurred from one sample to the next. The second was p-cresol (or para-cresol), a clear diaper-smelling liquid that would act as an internal standard, or control, to verify the equipment's operation. He needed to add these two solutions to the bile before he could undertake the actual analysis. However, he'd combine them in another container so that the vial of evidence bile remained intact.

With a small glass dropper, he extracted 20 microliters, the size of a water droplet, of bile from the first vial and squirted the droplet into a tiny microcentrifuge tube. He wanted enough of the bile so that its acids would show up if they were there. He then added 1 milliliter of methanol (to prevent cross-contamination of samples) and 30 microliters of p-cresol (as a control), capped off the tube, and labeled it. He and Shafer repeated the same meticulous preparation process for bile from each of the evidence gallbladders. The prepared samples would be used for both the HPLC and TLC tests.

When they'd completed several samples, Espinoza put the tubes in the centrifuge and flipped the switch. The machine hummed steadily as the tubes spun in a blurry circle. He waited a minute to guarantee adequate mixing and then stopped the instrument to exchange the tubes for another set.

When he'd blended all the samples, he carried them to the adjoining computer room, where he slotted the first tray into the corner of the HPLC machine. The innocuous gray instrument looked more like a set of large plastic blocks stacked on top of each other than a sophisticated piece of equipment. He opened the top and poured in the solutions needed to make it run: potassium phosphate (KH_2PO_4) to act as a buffer and pure, HPLC-grade water. The physical setup complete, he stepped in front of the computer to give the machine its instructions. Meticulously, he punched in a file name, set the flow rate and other parameters, and hit enter.

The machine whirred as the computer's commands started the mechanical arm, which grasped the first vial, inserted a tiny needle through the cap, and sucked up the solution. As the gripper moved out of the way, Espinoza watched the needle insert itself into an injection port. From there, the machine would combine the sample with the buffer and water and pump the new solution through an M. C. Escher–like system of valves and tubes until, fifteen minutes later, it would "decant" the dissolved solution through a thin column. Finally, a diode array detector would measure the ultraviolet (UV) spectrum of the sample and, from that, determine how long it took for each of the sample's components to move through the column, with the heavier, thicker acids taking longer. The computer would take this information and create a chromatogram, or picture, of the chemical profile, which Espinoza would read to see if the sample contained the unique bear bile acids. The instrument performed a separate operation for each sample and, before starting the next, would flush itself out to ensure no contamination.

Espinoza checked the machine and, confident it was working properly, returned to the lab to prepare the next round of bile.

Six hours later, Espinoza checked on the HPLC just as the machine's final clicks signaled the end of the analysis. He removed the samples and printed the chromatograms while Shafer set up the next group.

Back in his office, he laid the graphs across his desk. Reminiscent of a graph of an EKG heart monitor, the black-and-white printouts showed time (in minutes) across the horizontal bottom axis while the left-hand vertical y-axis exhibited measures of absorbance units, which reflect how much compound passed in front of the detector. While the bulk of the graph lines were fairly flat and fluctuated along the bottom, he was looking for three tall, fairly sharp peaks that would correspond to levels of particular bile acids.

Espinoza gazed at the first sample of the *known* bear bile and studied the chromatogram's peaks and troughs. Each indicated either the presence or absence of particular chemicals.

The first profile showed a peak for the p-cresol, the internal control he'd added to confirm that the machine itself worked properly. Good. Each chromatogram should have that.

His eye quickly located three additional peaks—one for each of the distinctive bear bile acids, with the dominant one being ursodeoxycholic acid (the others were chenodeoxycholic acid and cholic acid). Perfect. Now he just had to compare this with the profiles from the evidence samples.

He laid the profile from the first of Harrison's gallbladders just below the chromatogram from the bear. It, too, showed a spike for p-cresol but after that, the three additional peaks of bear bile were missing, replaced instead by a steplike series of six different peaks.

Expecting the next sample to show the pattern, he switched graphs but still the distinctive peaks were missing.

Again and again, the graphs for the evidence gallbladders showed initial spikes but then gave no indication that the samples contained bear bile acids. While all of the 182 exhibited the six peaks resembling bile acids, none of them looked anything like the three distinctive peaks of the known bear galls.

Though the HPLC had not produced the results he had expected, Espinoza figured that the more sensitive TLC might provide them. He put the same prepared samples on the counter near a box of TLC plates. He opened the carton and picked up one of the 8X8-inch glass squares by its edge, careful to keep his hands from touching the white silica gel coating painted on one side. Similar to HPLC, TLC separates mixtures and creates a picture of the chemicals from the different rate of their movement in an aqueous solution. This time, however, the picture would appear on the plate itself.

Espinoza set the plate on the counter and, with a fine-lead mechanical pencil and ruler, drew a straight line across the top and bottom. Measuring one and a half centimeters in from the edge, he made a small mark and, from there, made small dashes every centimeter until the end. These would be the starting points where he'd drop, or "spot," beads of the evidence solutions.

He finished scoring the plate, organized the equipment he'd need, and opened the cap of the first tube: the bear bile standard. He'd use the same evidence solutions he'd already prepared, only this time he wouldn't dissolve them further as he had in the HPLC process.

With a small, tapered glass dropper called a Pasteur pipetter, he sucked in the solution from the vial and squeezed it gently over the TLC plate to drop a small amount of liquid on the first dash.

He waited a minute for the spot to dry and added a second drop on top of the first to concentrate the solution. He repeated the process several times until he'd put two microliters, the size of a small water droplet, on that same spot.

He moved to the evidence samples, taking the next hour to concentrate eighteen of them on each of the remaining dashes, and finished with a sample of known bear bile.

When dry, the prepared TLC plate looked like it did when he'd started, only the pencil marks showed. He just needed to process the plate, like a photograph, to see the picture or chemical profile.

A TLC plate works like dumping a mixture of basketballs and Ping-Pong balls into a flowing creek. The big balls hit rocks and each other and are delayed, while the smaller balls flow easily with the water. For an observer downstream, the mixture of balls would separate into two distinct clumps. On the TLC plate, the liquid would flow up the plate, leaving tiny spots higher or lower depending on their molecular size. Smaller, faster chemicals, like ursodeoxycholic acid, would separate from the other bile acids and appear higher up, making it easy to identify them as samples from bear.[14]

Espinoza pulled out a developing tank, a Pyrex square about a foot around, and poured in 30 milliliters of chloroform, 4 milliliters of acetic acid, 30 milliliters of isopropyl alcohol, and 1 milliliter of the pure HPLC-grade water. With a glass rod, he stirred the mixture and moved the tank to the side to sit undisturbed for the next few hours.

When the solution had settled, Espinoza lowered the prepared TLC plate into the container and leaned its top end against the side. While the solvent didn't go up very high, just 3 millimeters, over time capillary action would absorb it and push it evenly up the plate. Espinoza put on the lid and turned to the next group of samples while he waited.

About two and a half hours later, Espinoza checked the plate and saw that the solution had worked its way to the top line. He took it out and positioned it upright in a cardboard box.

Now for the noisiest part: the "hair dryer from hell."

He plugged in the twenty-dollar high-powered appliance and pointed it at the glass. Ten minutes later, with the plate completely dry, he stuck it back in the developer for a second round. When the solvent reached the top line, he removed the plate and dried it again.

At last, the time had arrived for his favorite task: magician.

With a slight flourish, he misted the plate with glass sprayers, first with a 20 percent sulfuric acid solution and then with a 3.5 percent phosphomolybdic acid solution. Then, picking it up by the edges, he transferred the plate to a warm hot plate. To make sure the heat didn't concentrate in any one place, he slid it around constantly and watched smudges appear and slowly darken until, a couple minutes later, they'd developed fully.

The process had yellowed the white gel covering the square TLC plate, and rows of small and large, up to about half an inch, blue-black splotches now dotted the glass. The spots were neatly organized along the lines that he'd drawn earlier. The distance of the marks relative to the top of the plate told him if an evidence sample contained the bear acids. Similar to the HPLC, the first and last samples for the TLC procedure, the bear standards, showed clear patterns for the species. But the evidence samples, while also revealing a striking pattern, looked nothing like those of the bear standards.

Again, the results puzzled Espinoza.

Harrison had been so certain the gallbladders came from bear that Espinoza wondered if the tests might be faulty.

He called Hagey to go over the procedure and step-by-step they reviewed what the forensic scientist had done.

Hagey confirmed that Espinoza and his assistant had done everything perfectly. They *had* picked up the bear standards. And Hagey recognized the pattern of the evidence samples as pig. The results proved that the tests weren't faulty, but the gallbladders were. They were from pigs, not bears.

Now confident in the methodology but surprised by the results, Espinoza did the only thing he could do: plow ahead. The scientist wasn't disappointed. While deeply invested in the lab's overarching mission of protecting wildlife, when it came to the work he didn't care what the results showed—just that they were accurate.

Maybe some of the other samples would be those of bear.

Espinoza grimaced and called up the Criminalistics Examination Report for Harrison's case on his computer. He typed in the date—September 24, 1990—and keyed in the particulars for this case. In the main section, he summarized his conclusions: "All bile samples extracted from the evidence gallbladders did not contain the bile salt *Ursodeoxycholyl taurine* [UDC] which is consistent with belonging to the *Ursus* genus. Therefore, all the 182 gallbladders analyzed *are not bear gallbladders.*"[15]

Harrison wouldn't like the conclusion but Espinoza wasn't concerned. He couldn't change the results, nor would he want to. They were what they were. As a scientist, Espinoza focused solely on analyzing the evidence.

Like everyone at the lab, he remained indifferent to the outcome. The scientists' disinterest translated into a purposeful lack of awareness of the legal results of their cases. Unless called to testify, they rarely followed a case or even knew what happened with a suspect.

Forensic science has no agenda. It can just as easily prove someone innocent as guilty. As lab director Ken Goddard explained, "We don't want the scientist to get emotionally involved. We're not advocates. We don't try to help the prosecution. We simply answer investigative questions."[16]

By design, the lab fastidiously maintains its objectivity. Its scientists receive only the agent's request for examination of evidence, which describes the item and the type of analysis needed, such as species identification. The examiners don't see the investigative reports. They don't know the name of the suspect or the circumstances of the case. Without those details, they can't make assumptions about what their results mean even if they want to, which they don't. They can only assess what the evidence actually shows.

The credibility of the lab's analysis comes from its neutrality. Both sides, the defense and the prosecution, trust it because of the lab's deserved reputation for remaining unbiased. This impartiality makes the science so powerful that in nine out of ten cases the defense's legal team has decided not to challenge the lab's results. Indeed, from fiscal years 2003 through 2005, the lab testified in only 2.4 percent of its cases.[17] Most of the time, suspects pleaded out.

While that didn't happen in this case, the determination that Weston's gallbladders were not from bear and that he was not culpable simply underscored the lab's evenhandedness—and that deepened all-around confidence in its results.

Espinoza picked up the phone and told Harrison the results. The agent listened with surprise and dismay. Without forensic proof that Weston sold bear gallbladders, they had little against him. Selling gallbladders from other animals was perfectly legal. With little choice, the assistant U.S. attorney in Denver dropped the remaining wire- and mail-fraud charges against Weston so that, in the end, the dealer went free.

Weston's case illustrates how the prosecution of animal parts traffickers depends on the lab's ability to identify the origin of the product sold as a protected species. It doesn't matter if the dealer is duped. Without proof that the item came from a species whose trade is legally restricted or banned, prosecutors have nothing. And without a good shot at winning, wildlife agents, too, are hamstrung. They need the hammer of convictions that comes from the lab's species identification. Otherwise, they cannot enforce the law.

CHAPTER SIX

The Impact of Bear Investigation

Over the coming months, Harrison's case haunted Espinoza. Not because it had shown Weston to be innocent, but because the scientist wondered if a court would have ultimately accepted the validity of the identification process he used if they had proven the gallbladders were from bear.

Before the courts legitimized the protocol as a sound and authoritative way to identify the source of gallbladders, it had to be accepted by the scientific community. For that, it needed to be vetted further under a range of circumstances. The lab would have to establish that the methodology worked for gallbladders from known and unknown specimens, for species aside from bear, and for different structures, such as dried, frozen, and fresh organs and bile processed into crystals, powder, or other forms.

Beginning in 1990, after he'd finished analyzing Weston's gallbladders, Espinoza started to fill that information gap. He contacted everyone he could think of who might come across bear parts in their line of work, from FWS officers to state wildlife agencies and zoos, and begged them to donate their bear gallbladders to the lab.

To prove that a bear's bile acids were unique and that the TLC and HPLC tests detected the levels accurately and consistently, he tested as many known bear gallbladders as he could and compared the results with those from other species. Even though Espinoza had no bear gallbladder case pending, he pursued this data-gathering to help solve other violations. Often, when a case such as this one promises to be a recurring problem, the lab takes it on as a research project of sorts, which its scientists work at until they develop a protocol for future cases.

For example, when demand for caviar, the dissolution of the Soviet Union, and the resulting breakdown in the regulation of the caviar trade spurred overfishing of Caspian Sea sturgeon in the late 1990s, which contributed to a precipitous decline in many species and prompted their placement (in April 1998) on CITES Appendix II, the lab anticipated the imposition of new regulations to protect the fish and by 1998 had developed a DNA test to identify the various species. While similar genetic testing techniques had already been developed by researchers at the American Museum of Natural History in New York, the lab came up with its own because it could only use the existing technique by paying royalties on its patented parts. Paying royalties wasn't feasible because the lab needed a tool it could share freely with federal, state, and foreign enforcement agencies. The lab's DNA test for sturgeon resulted in convictions against numerous illegal caviar dealers. These include many who circumvented the prohibitions, like Mariusz Chomicz, the president of a caviar company in Poland who in 2004 was sentenced to thirty months in jail for paying couriers to smuggle caviar-filled suitcases into the United States without CITES certificates;[1] Viktor Tsimbal, president of Beluga Caviar, who had a similar scheme and in 2002 pleaded guilty to selling the protected roe under false labels;[2] and Grigori Oudovenko, a then thirty-nine-year-old Russian citizen and president of MNA Atlantic, a caviar exporting firm with offices in New York, Moscow, and St. Petersburg, who pleaded guilty in 2001 for attempting to smuggle 1,700 pounds of caviar worth $2.5 million in mislabeled containers into the United States.[3]

Little by little, samples of bear parts from a wide variety of sources trickled into the lab. The task of acquiring and confirming reference samples is one of the most vital parts of the wildlife forensics lab's work. Because most of its victims come to the lab as unidentifiable parts, such as a carved figurine, a purse, shawl, or powdered medicine, the lab can't rely on the commonly accepted species-defining characteristics, like an animal's appearance, sound, movement, diet, or habitat. Rather, it must establish other criteria.

To find these distinctive traits, the lab uses samples from known animals, called standards, as the basis for comparison. However, a single sample won't do. The characteristics of the parts of a single species can vary by gender or age. Feathers on juvenile eagles differ significantly from their adult coloration, and the plumage of male birds often diverges from that of females. Geography and diet also contribute to variations of certain traits. The tone of North American black bear fur fluctuates according to where the bear lives, with those from the open plains of the American west tending to be more cinnamon-colored and those from deeply forested areas in the eastern United States tending to be darker and blacker.

Similarly, the organs of the eight bear species might differ. For all Espinoza knew, gallbladders from grizzly, polar, Asiatic, and black bears could have diverse chemical or other characteristics. Or variation in the organs might occur between different ages, genders, or locations of the same species. For the comparisons to be convincing, Espinoza needed a lot of specimens. Not only that, but he had to know a lot about them—the species, age, gender, location, and the like—so that he could recognize any unique traits. Once the lab had received a sufficient number of standards, Espinoza would compare them to confirm whether *all* bear gallbladders had distinctive bile acids.

As the samples arrived, Espinoza and his assistant cataloged them. FWS special agent Ed Wickersham sent thirteen bear gallbladders, a researcher at the University of California–Davis sent five, and little by little the lab's menagerie of bear gallbladders grew. Each was accompanied by as detailed a description as possible about the animal it came from and where and how it had been obtained. Jim Wolfe from Alaska's Department of Public Safety's Scientific Crime Detection Laboratory sent muscle tissue, gallbladders, and hair from male and female brown bear cubs born early in 1990 and killed in October of that year in Alaska's Matanuska Valley—the cubs had been sent to him for postmortem exams. He also sent a jaw muscle from a male polar bear from Point Lay killed on December 8, 1990, after eating part of a villager.[4] (The lab would use the jaw muscle to build its database of bear DNA.) All of these samples were critical for the lab's scientists because without them, they would not be able to discern why specimens might differ.

Many contributors, like Chris Servheen, FWS's Grizzly Bear Recovery coordinator and co-chairman of the World Conservation Union's Species Survival Commission (IUCN/SSC) Bear Specialist Group, sent unconfirmed specimens, including both gallbladders being sold as bear and traditional Chinese medicines purporting to contain bear bile from Asian and North American markets, to the lab in addition to known bear gallbladders. These unknown samples would later prove useful for assessing why Harrison and Weston had been hoodwinked.

By late 1991, the lab had collected over three hundred known gallbladder specimens from a host of bear species from North America, Canada, Asia, and Russia.

Now to prove the protocol worked.

Espinoza and his assistant experimented with two other methods to detect the bear bile acids, but neither adequately characterized the species of an "unknown" bile sample. Gas chromatography-mass spectrometry (GC-MS) required manipulation of the sample, which could alter it, and Fourier transform infrared (FTIR) spectroscopy failed to separate individual molecules. That meant FTIR spectroscopy could only determine when a group of samples exhibited a particular pattern and not an *individual* one—a "must" for any forensic species identification. The scientists turned back to their protocol and demonstrated that together the HPLC and TLC processes consistently detected bear bile acids in any form.

With confirmation of their methodology in hand, the scientists next compared the known bear samples with gallbladders from other species to show the uniqueness of a bear's bile acid levels. The lab often searches for distinctive traits possessed only by a single species. For elephant ivory, Espinoza and his colleague Mary-Jacque Mann had homed in on the fine, curved lines radiating out from the center sections of the tusks. For rhinoceros horn, they had discovered that the wavelengths at which the "glue," or chemical binder, that holds the keratin fibrils together absorbed infrared light had a unique pattern that produced an idiosyncratic "fingerprint." For bear bile, Espinoza looked to the acid levels.

The scientist put out another call to federal and state wildlife agen-

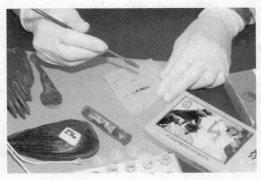

Analyzing traditional Asian medicines. *(Courtesy of U.S. Fish and Wildlife Service Forensics Laboratory)*

cies, zoos, and others who might have access to gallbladders, but this time asked for a variety of species. Again, organs trickled in. Soon, still during 1991, he had over five hundred from an array of animals— everything from pigs and cows to raccoons.

Comparing the gallbladders from bears to these other species, the scientists proved that the bear family (*Ursidae*) contained unique levels of three bile acids: ursodeoxycholic acid, chenodeoxycholic acid, and cholic acid.

No other species had the same pattern.

While the lab had verified both its methodology and the distinctiveness of bear bile acid levels, one puzzle remained: Why had Harrison and Weston both believed they'd been trading bear gallbladders when, in fact, they'd come from pig?

Maybe fraud was commonplace?

The lab's research into species identification of bile expanded into determining the amount of fraud in the marketplace. Knowing the extent of "fake" bear gallbladders would alert investigators to the possibility of deficient evidence and prompt them to ensure they collected sufficient proof of a crime. Espinoza and his assistant, Jo Ann Shafer, employed the bear bile identification protocol on the unknown specimens of gallbladders from Asian and North American traditional Chinese medicine markets that had been sent along with the known specimens.

By January 1992, they had the results. While 96 percent of the unknown gallbladders collected from Canadian markets were real (from bear), in the United States only 18 percent came from bear, and in Asia only 2 percent. The rest came from pigs.

Illegal traffickers were going to slaughterhouses, buying domestic pig gallbladders, and selling them as bear gallbladders. At a cost of about two dollars for a pig gallbladder, and anywhere from $150 to $5,000 for a bear's, the huge profits provided an irresistible incentive for substitution. Weston may have knowingly swapped the gallbladders, or maybe not. Most dealers probably benefited from the con. From their perspective, selling pig gallbladders as that from bears was a good way to make an extra buck. But now Espinoza would expect it. He wouldn't doubt his results.

Weston's case intersected with Olsen's case against Kim in Canada, and the work Espinoza had done gave Canadian prosecutors the evidence they needed to take Kim to trial. Kim's trial would be the protocol's first legal test, whereby the court would examine it in depth and officially establish its validity. That would make it a recognized and acceptable process to identify the origin of gallbladders in hundreds of future investigations.

In April 1994, Espinoza testified against bear parts dealer Sang Ho Kim in British Columbia's provincial court. After a morning spent qualifying as an expert witness, Espinoza explained the protocol. He started as he always did, by walking step-by-step through the science.

Pointing to a color-coded schematic of a bear on a metal stand in front, Espinoza led the court in "Bile 101" and explained that, of all the species tested, only bear had uniquely high levels of three specific bile acids.[5]

Next, he compared a chromatogram from a bear's gallbladder with one from a pig's.

"Anybody can look at them and see that they have a different profile," the scientist said.

The dissimilarities were obvious.

The scientist then described the testing procedures and presented his results: sixty-three of Kim's gallbladders were bear and the remaining twenty-three were from something else, likely pig.

With Espinoza's evidence-in-chief finished, Kim's defense attorney, George Wool, took over. An astute investigator and former sergeant in the commercial crimes section of the Royal Canadian Mounted Police (Canada's equivalent to the Federal Bureau of Investigation in the United States), he had a reputation for aggressively contesting every small detail of a case, one that he validated during his cross-examination.

Wool began by implying that the pig organs might have tainted the bear gallbladders when Conservation Officer Olsen sent *all* the evidence gallbladders in a single container to the lab.

That would invalidate the results, he argued.

Espinoza was unruffled. In an even, deliberate voice, he rebutted the implication by noting he'd cut into the bile sacs to extract the acids from the middle so that "we are assured that the source is not contaminated from the exterior environment." The scientist further explained that the tests would have picked up any contamination by exhibiting "overlappings of peaks from two different sources" in the chromatograms.

Unsatisfied, Wool grilled Espinoza on the chance the samples might have mixed during the analysis. But Espinoza remained unruffled. The scientist bluntly said that the machine automatically washed itself for five minutes between samples to prevent cross-contamination. And contrary to the defense attorney's hypothesis, the readout could not have been faulty because of the controls and standards.

"The controls and standards that are run with every batch of evidence tell us that the instrument is performing satisfactorily," Espinoza explained.

The cross-examination persisted for hours in this cat-and-mouse fashion, with Wool attempting to cast doubt over Espinoza's technique and Espinoza matter-of-factly squashing each intimation.

Finally, Wool had nothing left to ask.

Over the next year, Crown Counsel Jim MacAulay continued to prosecute the case and called on conservation officers Ralph Krenz and Rod Olsen, among others, to testify. In November 1995, the judge found Kim guilty of eleven of the twelve counts against him.[6]

At the end of the day, it was Espinoza's testimony that clinched the verdict. The day-long interrogation of the scientist had uncovered no flaws in his technique. Yet it had a second impact. Not only did it prove the case against Kim, but it validated the methodology itself and established a legally accepted way of identifying bear gallbladders.

About two months later, in mid-January 1996, Kim's sentencing took place. Crown Counsel MacAulay argued for a tough penalty. The prosecutor declared that Kim knew the law but chose to circumvent it. Worse, he did it for profit, as evidenced by the entrepreneur's brisk business and the almost C$20,000 (US$15,000) stockpile of bear parts at his house.

While Canada had a healthy population of black bears, commercialization of their parts could quickly change that if it's unregulated. MacAulay submitted a written statement from Chris Servheen that asserted unregulated "commercialization of wildlife has been a contributing factor in the reduction and loss of many wildlife species."[7]

In North America during the early 1900s, unregulated commercial activity decimated populations of ducks killed for meat, egrets for their tail plumes, and beaver for their fur. In many areas, elk and deer numbers also dropped to an all-time low due to selling their parts for profit. On the Great Plains, the commercial killing of tens of millions of bison for their hides nearly wiped them out as a wild species in less than forty years. More recently, in the 1970s and 1980s, elephant populations throughout Africa were depleted by Asian demand for ivory, and by the early 1990s (the time of Kim's trial), populations of both rhinoceros and Siberian tigers were on the verge of extinction due to demand for their parts for traditional Chinese medicine. When profits were available, people sought them out despite any laws to the contrary.

MacAulay contended that action was needed even though the population of black bears was currently healthy. With potential profits from illicit trade in bear parts nearly equaling that of illegal drugs, some legal opportunities for trade, limited fines, and minimal risk of jail time made selling bear parts particularly attractive.

In all probability, the low risk meant that the illegal bear parts trade would increase in North America. With wild Asian bears estimated to decline by 20 percent over the next decade, North America would soon be one of the only places left in the world where wild bear gallbladders could be collected. At the same time, demand for bear gallbladders and bile products was growing because of the increased personal wealth in those countries with strong cultural belief systems in traditional Asian medicine. Given the enormous number of users of traditional Chinese medicine worldwide, demand would continue to fuel the illegal bear parts trade unless both law enforcement and legal penalties were stepped up to limit it.

MacAulay pleaded that Kim receive a penalty severe enough to deter other poachers and traffickers, saying "the fine must not be a license fee for illegal activities."[8] He recommended jail and a C$40,000 to C$50,000 (US$30,000 to US$36,000) fine.

The judge fined Kim C$10,400 (US$7,600), the highest penalty in British Columbia to that date for a bear parts case. Like the bear identification protocol, the justification for action based on a future threat to a species' sustainability from its unregulated commercialization had its critical test in Kim's case—and won.

Yet despite the large fine, disappointment ran high as many observers feared the sentence wasn't enough of a deterrent. A *Vancouver Province* editorial noted, "We're still waiting for that one tough court sentence to send out the message that B.C. is serious about illegal trading in bear parts. Last week's sentence of $10,400 against a Surrey man doesn't cut it."[9] Environmentalists echoed that frustration and lobbied for more significant consequences. Though the profits available from illegally trading wildlife were high, the penalties if and when they were assessed often amounted to almost nothing.

Kim's case, and the others from Olsen's Operation Ice Bear investigation into bear gallbladder trafficking, had two major impacts in British Columbia. First, in the future, the unregulated commercialization rationale used in these cases would hold legal sway so that MacAulay and other environmental Crown Counsels could convict other dealers trafficking bear bile, sturgeon (caviar), and eagles (feathers). It allowed a precautionary approach to law enforcement and pursuit of cases involving species not currently endangered.

These cases also had another major impact: changing the law. As part of a series of trafficking schemes uncovered by Olsen's Operation Ice Bear, Kim's case raised awareness within the government about bear gall trafficking. Public consciousness was also raised when the media published several exposés on the trade, including an extensive front-page story on "bears on the brink" in the early 1990s in the *Vancouver Province* newspaper.

In response, British Columbia's environment minister John Cashore, who was sympathetic to the bears' plight, followed the Conservation Officer Service's recommendation to make the trade illegal. Olsen and his colleague Mark Hayden drafted the wording and in 1993 British Columbia adopted a new regulation making it illegal to possess, import, or sell bear gallbladders and their derivatives.

This modification was one of the rare instances when a wildlife enforcement operation changed the law. But, more important, by conforming to the same laws as its neighbors, the province removed a legal loophole for smugglers and eliminated its allure as a safe haven for dealers.

In the international arena, the number of cases like Weston's and Kim's prompted a major shift in the regulatory system. As these investigations showed, the decimation of wild Asian black bears had encouraged trade in gallbladders from North American black bears. As a result, environmental groups and animal rights advocates pressured the parties of the Convention on International Trade of Endangered

Species of Wild Fauna and Flora (CITES), the main global agreement to regulate international trade in listed wildlife species, to close the legal loophole that allowed for the substitution by listing North American black bears.

Bear gallbladders fall into a confusing legal class because trade in some places and in some species (like North American black bears or farmed Asian black bears) is allowed. The CITES parties addressed some of this inconsistency when they took up the bear's cause at its March 1992 Eighth Conference of Parties in Kyoto, Japan.

Adopted in 1973, CITES is a legally binding agreement (currently among 174 signatory nations, or Parties) that regulates international trade in listed wildlife and plant species in order to prevent or address their overexploitation and illegal trade. In March 1992, however, CITES had only 112 signatories, with key bear-parts-consuming countries, notably the Republic of Korea and Vietnam, joining later (in 1993 and 1994, respectively). Environmental organizations, academics, and government officials often consider CITES possibly the most effective environmental agreement to date because it relies on a sound scientific process to decide whether to include, remove, and recategorize species under protection and also maintains clear enforcement mechanisms.

The Convention has several categories of protection. The most restrictive level, Appendix I, prohibits trade that is primarily for commercial purposes and includes those imperiled species that are, or may be, affected by trade. All Asian bear species—including the Asiatic black bear (or moon bear), the brown bear, sun bear, sloth bear, and giant panda—are included in Appendix I. Other species, including those not yet threatened with extinction but which may become so without trade regulations, fall under Appendix II, which limits and controls trade by requiring traders to have a permit for exports. The lowest level of protection, Appendix III, applies when a country seeks international cooperation to enforce its national restrictions regarding a species. Canada sought this for its black bear populations so that, as of September 18, 1991, its black bears were listed under Appendix III and required a (Canadian) permit for export.

Protections for CITES-listed species are implemented and enforced through the signatory nations' domestic legislation. The United States, for example, implements CITES protections largely through the Endangered Species Act (ESA), which preserves the habitats of endangered species and prohibits their possession, capture, and sale (without permits), and the Lacey Act, which forbids possession or sale of wildlife and plants taken, possessed, or sold in violation of an underlying federal, state, tribal, or foreign law.

Just as the Seventh Conference of Parties in 1989 in Lausanne, Switzerland, that transferred African elephants to Appendix I (and in effect temporarily banned commercial trade in elephant ivory) was a pivotal moment for elephants, this 1992 CITES meeting proved to be a watershed moment for North American black bears. After much heated debate, the Parties agreed that in order to improve the protection of the endangered Asian bear species, they would restrict trade in North American black bears under Appendix II as a look-alike species.

The CITES intention was to protect Asian bears, but in order to do so they also had to protect North American black bears. Asian bears couldn't be protected without restricting trade in their substitute because the similarity of the two species' gallbladders made it difficult to enforce existing commercial trade bans on the Appendix I–listed Asian bears. Smugglers evaded the bans by claiming their products came from the legally allowed North American black bears rather than from the restricted species. The listing of North American black bears under Appendix II aimed to prevent that deception by requiring documentation for North American black bear parts (while still allowing their sale). This way, sellers would have to prove their organs' species.

While environmentalists viewed it as clearly a key victory, the CITES Appendix II listing of North American black bears was only a first step. National legislation and enforcement were still needed to implement it.

Until 1997, not much happened. But a broad consensus on the issue did grow among both supplying and consuming nations. So much so that at the June 1997 Tenth CITES Conference of Parties in Harare, Zimbabwe, the Parties unanimously and without debate adopted a resolution on the "Conservation of and Trade in Bears."[10] The issue had gathered so much support that the United States, which had vehemently opposed the 1992 listing, co-authored the resolution.

The 1997 resolution reiterated CITES's commitment to protecting bears by stopping the illegal bear parts trade and urged Parties "to take immediate action in order to demonstrably reduce the illegal trade in bear parts and derivatives" by, among other actions, "confirming, adopting or improving their national legislation to control the import and export of bear parts and derivatives."[11]

Canada did not establish a national prohibition on trade in bear gallbladders, but in May 1996 it enacted the federal Wild Animal and Plant Protection and Regulation of International and Interprovincial Trade Act (WAPPRIITA) to prohibit the transportation of illegally obtained, possessed, or distributed wildlife or its parts between provinces and territories or between Canada and other countries (similar to the Lacey Act's provisions in the United States).

In 1998, the United States renewed efforts to pass national legislation (which was first introduced in 1992 but only related to black bears). Dubbed the Bear Protection Act, it aimed to prohibit all trade in bear parts rather than leave it up to the states. The bill's sponsor, Senator Mitch McConnell (R.-Ky.), told his colleagues on the Senate Environment and Public Works Committee at a July 7, 1998, hearing, "As long as a few states permit this action to go on, poaching for profit will continue."[12]

In the United States, the Bear Protection Act seemed like a reasonable law. It would establish a uniform prohibition on trade in bear viscera yet not prevent legal hunting or weaken existing state laws. However, it didn't pass. While it had significant bipartisan support in Congress, powerful legislators, in particular Representative Don Young (R.-Alaska), feared that it opened the door for a permanent ban on bear hunting. Each time a version of the bill came up, these opponents, together with many hunting organizations, pressured their colleagues either to stop the act from being put to a full vote or to vote against it. While the act passed in the U.S. Senate twice, it never passed in the U.S. House of Representatives.

In 2008, the Bear Protection Act (H.R. 5534) was again introduced in the U.S. House of Representatives. As before, this act would prohibit the trade of bear viscera and bear viscera products in both interstate and international trade. Yet the prospects for passage were negligible. At a March 11, 2008, hearing on the bill before the Subcommittee on Fisheries, Wildlife and Oceans of the House Committee on Natural Resources, both the FWS's chief of law enforcement, Benito Perez, and the president of the Association of Fish and Wildlife Agencies, Matt Hogan, opposed it, saying it would cost too much to implement, that it duplicated existing legal authority, and it unnecessarily intruded into state wildlife management authorities.

Others vehemently disagreed. Wayne Pacelle, president and chief executive officer of The Humane Society of the United States, testifying on behalf of the Bear Working Group of the Species Survival Network, Animals Asia, and Born Free USA, argued that persistence of the trade, as evidenced by the December 2007 arrest of a San Diego, California, bear gallbladder dealer, among others, necessitated harmonization of state laws. He argued that the legislation would not be a burden or cost money to implement but rather would be another tool that state and federal wildlife agents could use as they saw fit.

Interestingly, Ray Schoenke, president of the American Hunters and Shooters Association, a then two-year-old pro-hunting gun rights organization, and a former Washington Redskins football player, also supported the act. He contended it was narrowly crafted so that it would assist state and federal wildlife law enforcement efforts without "federalizing hunting, usurping lawful sportsmen's ability to hunt bears in accordance with state laws and regulations, or undermining the ability of state game agencies to otherwise manage their resident bear populations."[13]

However, once again, the bill never passed out of committee. The National Rifle Association (NRA), joined by other hunting organizations and the Association of Fish and Wildlife Agencies, sent a letter opposing the bill to every member of the House. With this pressure, the committee refrained from further action until it could be certain the bill had sufficient votes.

Whether Congress will recognize, as Canada already has, the threat unregulated commercialization poses to black bears despite a currently healthy population is anybody's guess. One noteworthy point is the strong commitment of Representative John Campbell (R.-Calif.), who is a co-sponsor of the bill and a passionate advocate for it. Coming from an avid hunter and NRA supporter, his backing may change the tide by demonstrating that the act would simply prevent poaching, the *illegal* killing of animals, and not stop legal hunting.

While the bill's prospects remain unclear, what is certain is that the need for uniform regulations still exists. Bear gallbladders and bile continue to be highly sought after commodities, and the legal market appears to facilitate and promote the illegal trade.[14]

• • •

Aside from the legal regime for bears, another area of significant controversy is the status of bear farms in Asia. The idea of farming instead of killing wildlife began in the early 1950s, when Chinese farmers harvested musk, a strong-smelling substance worth $40,000 per kilogram ($18,200 per pound) secreted by male musk deer and used to treat malaria, convulsions, and other ailments. In what it claimed was an effort to stop the poaching of Asian black bears, China opened its first bile milking operations in 1984 (following North Korea in 1980 and South Korea in 1983, and before Vietnam in 1993),[15] and these bears are now among the thirty wild species (including tigers) bred, caught, and kept in captivity for use in traditional Chinese medicine.[16]

The issues surrounding bear farms are twofold. First, the squalid conditions and unsafe medical practices were not only inhumane, they halved the lives of farmed bears compared to their wild brethren. In 1993, Jill Robinson, who was investigating bear farming practices on behalf of the International Fund for Animal Welfare (IFAW), exposed the inhumanity of the practice. Posing as a proper British tourist, Robinson infiltrated a Japanese tour group as it entered a bear farm in Zhuhai in China's Guangdong Province, one of hundreds across China, South Korea, and Vietnam.

Following the group toward the farm's breeding pits—the tour's main attraction—Robinson was horrified when the visitors teased the bears with fruit hung on fishing poles and laughed at the melee as the animals fought over the pitiful morsels. With everyone focused on the activity inside the pit, Robinson slipped away and found the milking facility at the bottom of a plain staircase.

Rows and rows of tiny cages, which would eventually become coffins for their moon bear prisoners, lined the dimly lit basement while strange popping vocalizations and an odor of stale urine filled the air. The bears inside looked as if they'd been subjected to medieval torture. Rusting catheters protruded from gaping wounds in the bears' bellies, and blood, bile, and pus seeped from the holes. Their canine teeth had been cut back. Many had three- to four-foot scars along their bodies or head wounds from bashing themselves against the bars in feeble attempts at mental stimulation. Some had missing paws. When Robinson crept close to the cages, their popping vocalizations got more frantic. "They clearly associated me with the painful bile extraction they had to endure twice a day," she recalled.[17]

The visit to what Robinson called "a torture chamber, a hell hole for animals"[18] exposed the cruel practice in the media and generated an international outcry against it by animal rights activists and environmental groups. In addition to protesting the appalling conditions and methods, these groups maintained that bear farms did more than harm the bears in captivity—they stimulated demand for bear bile by making it accessible to more people at lower prices.[19]

Reduced prices and wider availability expanded the overall market. According to the World Society for the Protection of Animals (WSPA), bear bile use increased tenfold over a twenty-five-year period, from 1,100 pounds (0.55 tons, or 500 kilograms) per year for traditional medicines in China in 1980 (before the farms) to between 8,800 and 11,000 pounds (4.4 to 5.5 tons, or 4,000 to 5,000 kilograms) per year worldwide for medicines and other uses in 2005.[20] Demand is met by illegal trafficking in wild bears and legally farming captive ones, and the pressure on each grows every year. As of the early 2000s, Asian

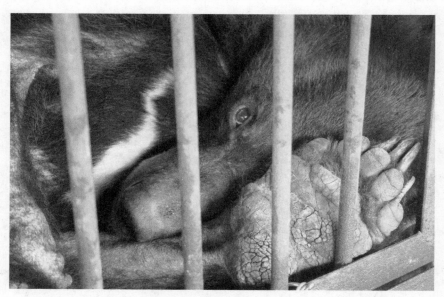

Asiatic black bear in cage at bear farm. *(Courtesy of Animals Asia Foundation)*

farms held over 11,000 bears, with 7,000 in China, 1,800 in South Korea, and 2,400 in Vietnam.[21]

The bear farm industry and its supporters argue that the practice, by providing bile for traditional medicines, prevents the killing of wild bears. According to one of China's senior wildlife officials, Wang Wei, deputy director of the Department of Wildlife Conservation under the State Forestry Administration, "If one black bear was raised for gall extraction, it means that 220 black bears could survive."[22] An official of Guanxian City, where a municipal bear farm was being established, explained, "Bear bile is so popular that if we cannot find an efficient way to produce it, people will shoot all the bears."[23]

Unfortunately, bear bile use has expanded beyond traditional medicine to a range of other products. While its former rarity and exorbitant cost used to mean practitioners turned to it only in the severest cases when other treatments had failed, now more people seek it out as a cure-all for every ailment.

Further, the shortage of bear bile that these farms supposedly fill is no longer in existence. The new sources of bile have created a surplus. As of 2005, bear bile supplies from farmed and wild sources exceeded demand from traditional medicine markets alone by about 4,400 pounds (2.2 tons, or 2,000 kilograms) per year, and as a result, that "excess" bile is now added to an array of "luxury" goods ranging from hemorrhoid creams to shampoos, wines, and vitamins.[24] Rather than dying to cure human diseases, bears are now being killed for garish consumer products for the wealthy.

Despite persistent and expanding markets, the efforts to reduce illegal trade in bear gallbladders and bile have resulted in several encouraging victories. North American black bear populations have remained healthy in most parts of the continent and dire predictions have not come to pass—yet. Notably, the CITES listing of North American black bears raised the profile of the issue and initiated the first series of legislative steps to remove this easy route for illegal smuggling.

In Asia, China and other countries have closed many of their bear farms and made their operations more humane. In July 2000, after seven years of intense negotiation and trust building, Animals Asia Foundation (Robinson's Hong Kong–based animal rights organization), the China Wildlife Conservation Association (CWCA) (part of the State Forestry Administration in Beijing), and the Sichuan Forestry Department signed an agreement to free five hundred captive bears. At a farm's closure, farmers would return their original license to Animals Asia and receive compensation for their bears. The government would then refrain from issuing new licenses. The arrangement was a significant step toward Animals Asia's ultimate goal of eliminating China's then (in 2000) 250 bear farms and freeing their 7,000 bears.

In October 2000, Animals Asia Foundation's Sichuan Long Qiao Black Bear Rescue Centre in Chengdu in China's Sichuan Province accepted its first three rescued bears. While many rescued bears died over the next seven years from liver cancer and other diseases resulting from their years of incarceration, by 2007, the $3 million sanctuary, which included a hospital, fenced-in living area, and twenty-seven-acre tract of bamboo forest, housed about two hundred bears from over forty closed farms, with more arriving every year.

While acknowledging the cruel methods used at some bear farms, China has also instituted a series of measures to improve conditions at remaining bear farms. These include the enactment of "interim provisions for a technical code of practice for raising black bears" that

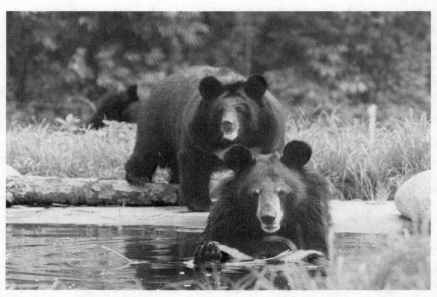

Rescued Asiatic black bears at sanctuary. *(Courtesy of Animals Asia Foundation)*

requires hygienic, painless bile extraction and regulates the methods and conditions for captivity and breeding, and the prosecution of offenders.[25]

Similar successes occurred in Vietnam. Since 1998, Animals Asia Foundation together with other nongovernmental organizations such as Education for Nature–Vietnam, Wildlife at Risk, and TRAFFIC, the international wildlife trade monitoring organization, encouraged the government to implement a law to make bear farming illegal. Also, in 2005 the Vietnamese government committed to the World Society for the Protection of Animals to phase out bear farming and signed an agreement with Animals Asia Foundation to rescue two hundred farmed bears in Hanoi, with the first ones arriving in October 2007.[26]

At the same July 2000 meeting when China agreed to free five hundred captive bears, Animals Asia, the China Wildlife Conservation Association, and the Sichuan Forestry Department also pledged to promote herbal and synthetic alternatives to bear bile. Though still in its nascent stages, a clear and growing movement among traditional Asian medicine practitioners exists toward replacing bear bile with herbal and other alternatives.

At the Third International Symposium on Trade in Bear parts, held in October 1999 in Seoul, South Korea, the president of the Practicing Pharmacists Association of Hong Kong, Scarlett Oi Lan Pong, noted that while bear gallbladders had effectively treated tumors and stomach and liver disease for over four hundred years, it was only one of more than sixty effective treatments. Pong observed, "If we remove bear gallbladder from the list of treatments for these symptoms, we certainly still have a lot of herbal products from which to choose."[27] A 1994 study by the Earth Care Society (Hong Kong) and the Association of Chinese Medicine and Philosophy confirmed this statement when it established the effectiveness of over fifty-four herbal alternatives to bear bile.

In addition, a joint campaign started in 1997 by the International Fund for Animal Welfare (IFAW), Animals Asia Foundation, and several traditional medicine associations in Hong Kong built a coalition of traders, consumers, and over five thousand doctors and traditional Asian medicine practitioners who pledged "not to use endangered species in any products [they] prescribe, sell or buy" and to replace them with herbal alternatives.[28]

A growing number of practitioners of traditional Chinese medicine now prescribe alternatives, in part because of their effectiveness and lower cost and in part because of their belief that the brutal means of obtaining bear bile—that is, either poaching endangered species or cruel farming methods—contradicts the underlying principle of traditional Asian medicine of maintaining harmony with nature. As Dr. Lo Yan Wo of the Hong Kong Chinese Herbalist Association put it: "Culture should not be used as an excuse for cruelty and in Traditional Chinese Medicine there are many alternatives to the use of these animals."[29] Taken together, these efforts demonstrate a growing movement in Asia toward replacing bear bile with other substances.

In some sense, a test of alternatives has already been done. Prior to the lab's 1992 revelation of the lack of bear bile in packaged TCM products, people weren't aware of the switch. They happily used the pig bile products and thought they worked; with that acceptance they indicated that bear bile was not always absolutely necessary.

Other manufactured traditional Chinese medicines, meaning the relatively recent business of prepackaged medicines manufactured by Chinese companies and not the hand-prepared ones mixed in apothecaries, have employed other animals as a critical ingredient and exhibited the same deceit.

The existence of widespread fraud in the "patented" traditional Chinese medicinal trade demonstrates the efficacy of the placebo effect and opens the door for alternatives to rare animal products. Espinoza compares the substitution to the consistent failure to find real tiger bone in patented Chinese medicines, like medicinal tea balls to musk-tiger bone plasters. Despite claims that these items contain bone from rare tigers, neither he nor his colleagues, including those at Scotland Yard and Environment Canada, have detected it. Of patented medicines purporting to contain deer musk, less than 0.5 percent in the United States actually did. In Hong Kong, less than 1.6 percent of patented deer musk medicines contain it and in Taiwan only 20 percent is real.[30] With these low percentages for a relatively abundant species, Espinoza expects the findings would be even more pronounced for rarer commodities, like tiger bone and rhino horn.

Despite these promising developments, however, alternatives and synthetics are "not accepted by everybody. . . . We need to face this," Dr.

Fan Zhiyong of China's CITES Management Authority noted.[31] For bears, that means alternatives will never satisfy demand for their gallbladders "any more than cubic zirconium [satisfied] the demand for diamonds."[32]

Sadly, recent signs in the international arena point to a possible deepening of the demand for bear bile, and a corresponding worsening of illegal trafficking and expansion of bear farming. China maintains that advanced techniques for extracting bile from live bears, such as tubes made of bear tissue, make the procedure painless,[33] although animal welfare advocates disagree. In 2006, China rejected the European Parliament's call for an immediate ban on the "cruel and uncivilized practice" of bear farming. It argued that bear bile remained an essential ingredient in traditional Chinese medicine with no viable substitute. This denial of the efficacy of alternatives may as well have been an endorsement of the use of bear bile.

Further evidence of China's lack of intention to reduce demand for rare wildlife parts used in traditional Chinese medicine is its position on tiger parts at the June 2007 CITES Conference of Parties, wherein it reasoned that the ban should be lifted.[34] China proposed legalizing the sales of tiger parts because of its effective enforcement and successful tiger farming efforts. Siberian tigers, with populations of between 300 and 400 individuals, are on the verge of extinction due, in large part, to their use in traditional Chinese medicine. Similarly, populations of all kinds of tigers in the wild have plummeted from 25,000 to 30,000 fifty years ago to about 5,000 now.[35]

At the 2007 CITES meeting, China said the 1993 ban on tiger parts trade failed to stop poaching, cost its economy almost four billion dollars, and blocked medical treatment for the poor. It contended that its five thousand captive-bred tigers could supply breeding stock for reintroduction into the wild and also offered an opportunity to reopen the tiger bone and fur market.[36] While the proposal was not accepted by the CITES Parties (they instead adopted a decision that "tigers should not be bred for trade in their parts and derivatives"[37]), China's efforts indicate their intention to continue and expand wildlife farming for commercial gain.

"It's a different definition of conservation," Don Reid, a World Wildlife Fund researcher, explained in the early 1990s. "For the Chinese, conservation has entirely a utilitarian end. That is, you need to make sure there are bears somewhere—not necessarily in the wild—in order for you to continue to have gall. But that's about as far as it goes."[38]

Given China's attempt to reopen the marketing of tiger parts from its farms, it seems like a natural step for China to actively promote bile from its bear farms. According to the deputy director-general for China's Department of Wildlife Conservation, Wang Wei, as of early 2006 China had sixty-eight bear farms with seven thousand bears.[39] That's in spite of promises to reduce the numbers. While the quantity of facilities declined, the amount of captive bears has remained unchanged from 2000 levels. This shows a broad shift away from many small-scale farms to fewer large ones housing greater numbers of animals, which may make them easier to regulate.

As Kurt Johnson, senior program officer for TRAFFIC USA in the early 1990s, said, "Bear farming might be laudable if it did take pressure off wild populations. But in the way it appears to be done in China, it's simply an agricultural practice."[40] Bear farms are money-making enterprises and, as such, have the goal of increasing sales and expanding markets.

According to a statement by China's vice minister of science and technology, Liu Yanhua, at the Second International Conference on the Modernization of Chinese Medicine held in Chengdu, China, in September 2005, China's pharmaceutical sector was worth almost $12 billion in 2004 and is the world's fastest growing, with its value expanding at 18 percent per year.[41] In just a decade, from the mid-1990s to mid-2000s, China's domestic demand for traditional medicines swelled 300 percent.[42] International demand also rose. In 2005, China exported $153 million worth of traditional Chinese medicine to Asia, Europe, and North America, a surge of 10 percent from the previous year.[43] That expansion will probably continue as China modernizes its industry and moves traditional medicine away from a localized system catering to its own people to one more widely accepted internationally. As part of that shift, the Chinese government designated traditional medicine production a strategic industry[44] and announced in April 2007 a fifteen-year plan to dedicate almost $130 million, five times the previous year's budget, to improve testing, expand clinical research, and develop globally recognized standards for treatments.[45]

Testing and research could validate the effectiveness of traditional Chinese medicines that employ rare and endangered species as a key ingredient, or it might show their lack of value and the efficacy of alternatives. Currently, no scientific evidence proves tiger bone is better than pig or goat bone to relieve joint pain, and some doctors have effectively substituted bone from the north China rat.[46] Even so, convincing Asian consumers about the efficacy of substitutes is an uphill task given their long-held use and cultural beliefs.

Many environmentalists and scientists, such as Chen Shilin, deputy director of the Institute of Medicinal Plant Development in the Chinese Academy of Medical Sciences, contend that traditional Chinese medicine hurts China's biodiversity and is a major factor threatening the extinction of species.[47] Worldwatch Institute notes that traditional Chinese medicine is a top conservation threat for Asia's bear, tiger, and rhinoceros populations, surpassing habitat loss.[48] According to the World Wildlife Fund, over the last twenty years, traditional Chinese medicine's growing popularity spurred poaching and illegal trade of threatened and endangered species to "crisis levels" and negated the progress made in establishing laws and nature reserves to protect these animals.[49]

To address overexploitation, China's State Forestry Administration and State Administration for Industry and Commerce introduced a labeling system in May 2003 that would "distinguish traditional medicine containing legal wildlife ingredients from those of unsustainable and illegal origin."[50] The lab's forensic identification techniques could help certify their legal origin and support this sustainable "branding." The government has also invested almost $4 million in research on alternatives to endangered species.[51] These efforts are the result of the 1999 pledge by Chinese officials, when traditional Chinese medicine sales worldwide were just $1 billion (less than a tenth of what they are today), to make the trade more sustainable.[52] These measures come at a time when China is investing even more heavily in expanding the industry, suggesting the possibility of conflicting policies.

While the idea of farming bears has merit, it must be done in a way that obtains the product without harming the animal, like shearing sheep, milking cows, or even dehorning rhinoceros. The question is: under what conditions can and should bear bile be milked in a humane way?

At the same time, the issues of what is an acceptable level of bear bile use, and if a mechanism can be developed to allow it in traditional medicine but prevent it from being used as a frivolous component in luxury products, should also be explored.

The solution to protecting bears and the interests of traditional Chinese medicine practitioners lies in keeping illegal trade low enough to ensure the continuation of the species—through harmonized laws and better enforcement—while simultaneously examining supplies and reducing demand through education and alternatives.

In the United States, the work of the FWS forensics lab helps convict violators. By proving that dealers illegally trade bear gallbladders for use in the traditional Asian medicine market, it brings to light the problem. That exposure has already helped change laws and reform bear farming practices. It can also help reduce demand for bear bile products and create support for substitutes.

The threat against bears continues. The inconsistency of state laws, the confusing legal status of different bear species in different locations, and the difficulties in telling the gallbladders of these protected bear species apart combine with high profits, low penalties, and underfunded and understaffed wildlife law enforcement agencies to make limiting the illicit trade difficult.

The bottom line is that bear galls are small, profitable, and easy to smuggle, and that bears are far from safe. Yet the lab's forensic support for enforcement makes illegal traders more vulnerable. They can no longer act with immunity—and that's good for the bears.

CHAPTER SEVEN

The Feather Artifacts

The young boy paddled in front of his father, at times ducking to avoid the thick foliage overhanging the narrow waterway. Like other Indian children in Brazil's Amazon Basin, the boy learned what he needed to survive in the rain forest from his parents and elders. He belonged to the Rikbatsa tribe, one of over two hundred distinct indigenous groups in the Amazon, each with different cultures and traditions: some were sedentary and practiced slash-and-burn agriculture, while others, like the Rikbatsa, were nomadic and moved from place to place to hunt and gather food.

The Rikbatsa, which means "the human beings," live on Brazil's Juruena River basin in the northwestern part of the state of Mato Grosso.[1] They are known as *canoeiros,* or canoe people, and capitalize on the intertwining paths of water for transportation and the surrounding fertile lands for agriculture.[2] Reputed to be fierce warriors, they were largely isolated until the late 1940s, when rubber gatherers arrived in their homelands. The contact with outsiders exposed them to diseases they'd never encountered, and their lack of immunity stirred epidemics that decimated their populations. Their numbers dropped from about 1,300 individuals at first contact to 300 in 1969, and then rebounded to about 1,000 today.[3]

The canoe floated silently down the river with an occasional splash the only indication it was there. The boy and his father listened to the sounds around them as a harsh, drawn-out screech rose above the forest's steady buzz of insects. The father focused on the sound, as if amplifying it by sheer will, and the boy mimicked his actions. The thick greenery of the rain forest hid the animals, so that they had to use their other senses—hearing and smell—to find them.

The hunt wasn't for enjoyment. The Rikbatsa needed the animals for food and for the raw materials to make tools, clothes, buildings, and adornments. They ate almost every animal available to them; birds, peccary (like a wild pig), white-tailed deer, agouti, tapir, coatis, pacas, armadillos, river otter, tayra, and most monkeys were all fair game.

Like many indigenous Indian tribes in the Amazon, the Rikbatsa's religious beliefs were intimately tied to the natural world. They donned feathers or other animal parts to take on the properties of a particular creature and thereby gain that species' strengths and insights.

They also believed that physical beings exchanged "souls." This basic principle tends to be constant across tribes, although the specifics differ. The Rikbatsa avoid hunting a white-haired ape called a night monkey because they believe their dead tribesmen might be reincarnated as that species. They also steer clear of killing jaguars and snakes because they might be the reincarnation of people who were evil in life and were now intent on transmitting their bad luck. Other indigenous groups, however, such as the Bororo, who live in Mato Grosso on the margins of the Xingu River, view jaguars not as wicked but as a source of strength, cunning, and a direct connection to the spirits. Jaguars play several roles in Bororo culture. At death, the Bororo believe, a person's soul moves into the body of certain animals, including the jaguar. As part of the subsequent funeral ritual, a man representing the deceased hunts a large cat and gives its skin to the dead person's relatives to guarantee vengeance over the supernatural entity that caused the death. In addition, jaguar teeth necklaces are worn as a status symbol by Bororo shamans.

The Rikbatsa Indian father looked up and squinted, as if by resolve he could adopt the harpy eagle's acute vision and render the trees transparent. The boy's gaze followed and picked out a glint of red as it flashed through the canopy just as a scarlet macaw dropped its tail for a landing. The birds preferred this unique area of riparian tropical forest bordering the edges of seasonally flooded river because it provides the greatest densities of their favorite nesting trees, such as the kapok (also known as ceiba, or silk cotton tree, *Ceiba pentandra*), bacurubu (*Schizolobium parahybum*), or danto (*Vatairea lundelli*).

With their striking red, yellow, and blue colors; long, narrow wings; and elongated, graduated tail that lets them fly long distances, scarlet macaws are probably the most magnificent and recognized bird in the parrot family. Because many of the seventeen macaw species need large tracts of pristine habitat to survive, researchers believe their status may provide an indication of the health of the rain forest.

Like other macaws, scarlet macaws are seed predators, meaning they eat and destroy seeds instead of eating just the fruit and dropping the seed or dispersing it far from the parent tree in their stool. Seed predators play an important role in the ecosystem by limiting the number of competing seeds and thus leaving more resources for successful germination of the remaining ones.

Scarlet macaws, with their long life span of forty to fifty years (and up to seventy-five years in captivity),[4] mate for life and have low reproduction rates that can't easily withstand overexploitation. They range across Central America and northern South America and, because they are described as common in parts of their range, are listed by IUCN's Red List as a species of least concern. However, their global population has not been quantified, and evidence suggests declining populations, partly due to fragmentation and loss of their habitat from deforestation, hunting for food and feathers, and capture to supply the North American and European pet trade. Consequently, scarlet macaws are listed under CITES Appendix I and protected throughout their range.

The boy reached for his bow and took an arrow from the quiver slung on his back in an action he'd watched his father make a hundred times before. The blunted arrow would prevent blood from damaging or soiling the feathers. It also meant he wouldn't kill the bird. The Rikbatsa raised several kinds of birds, including macaws, curassows, and chickens, among others, as a source of feathers for their artifacts. Once plucked, the feathers would regrow quickly, perhaps a week later, and often come in even brighter and bolder than before.

The plumes from this bird might go into any one of a number of adornments, each of which might be used in an important cultural ceremony, such as a rite of passage into adulthood, agricultural ceremony, or other special occasion. Many Amazonian Indian tribes used feathers in their body adornments, costumes, and implements as a central part of their rituals. The feathered full-body costumes and headdresses that sat hatlike with feathers spiking up to the sky or armbands that converted arms into wings transformed the wearers into giant birds and transported them into the spiritual realm.

Because of their spiritual significance, the decorations revealed a lot about the traditions and beliefs of the people who made them, and each artifact had its own story to tell. The Rikbatsa wear armbands and crowns, often with sprigs of red feathers on the top highlighted by black and white feathers behind and on the bottom as well as by bright yellow feathers, at many of their agricultural, naming, marriage, and other ceremonies; they tend to be part of the standard regalia. For the Hixkaryana people, a tribe of about five hundred who live in Brazil's Amazonas State near the Nhamunda River, their decorated hair tubes reflect the men's belief that their spiritual strength resides in their hair. They pull their long locks back into the feathered cylinders, so that the attached harpy eagle feathers dangle down their backs, to enhance their hair's power and better connect to the spiritual world.

In a larger sense, these stunning feathered artifacts represent the last vestiges of dying cultures. For many Brazilian indigenous groups, the opening of the rain forest to farming, logging, and mining is destroying the fragile ecosystem on which they depend and hastening their demise. When the Europeans first arrived, Brazil had over a thou-

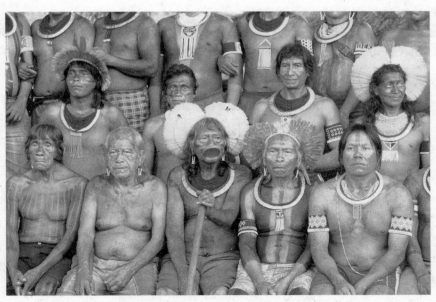

Brazilian Amazon Kayapó Indians wearing feathered body costumes.
(Courtesy of Cristina G. Mittermeier)

sand distinct indigenous Indian groups with a total population between 2 and 4 million people. Today, only 220 indigenous groups comprising about 370,000 individuals remain, with about 60 percent living in the Amazon.[5] Most tribes are small, like the Bororo and Rikbatsa, who each comprise about 1,000 people; others, like the Wayana with about 400 individuals in Brazil and the Ikpeng with 300, are minuscule.[6] As a result, the adornments have become "books" to store the living history of these ancient but disappearing cultures.

The bird flapped his wings to brake and stretched his feet down to grasp the branch below.

The limb bounced to accommodate the animal's weight and the boy and his father recognized the signal. Their quarry was near.

Throughout the Amazon, similar scenes of hunting, creating adornments, and performing rituals to mark life passages repeat themselves, as they have for thousands of years.

In Pará, Brazil, the Amazonian Indian Wayana-Aparai boys gather in the central plaza at dawn after spending hours in the forest with the shaman constructing elaborate headdresses and dance costumes. They'd decorated the adornments with bright macaw, toucan, and curassow feathers that had been carefully preserved in bamboo tubes and plaited baskets.[7] Their bellies were full. In preparation for the day ahead, they'd gorged themselves on food that their mothers had specially prepared as a parting gift. They needed the energy. It was the last food or drink they'd consume over the next twenty-four hours.

Adorned in their special attire, the boys dance in rhythmic movements that will carry them through the day and night while, nearby, the shaman and his aides prepare for the next part of the ceremony. Meticulously, they gulp mouthfuls of tobacco smoke and blow the intoxicating substance over hundreds of large wasps they'd collected earlier. As the fumes waft over the insects, the frenzy of flying slows until the creatures become comatose. With the wasps in this altered state, the shaman weaves about a hundred of them into a small, rectangular panel in the center of an elaborate feathered shield and repeats the process for each boy. By nightfall, he's ready.

One by one, the boys step forward. Their tired movements reveal their exhaustion from lack of nourishment and a day of nonstop dancing. The wasps, too, remain sleepy. That is, until the shaman wakes them by hitting the shields against a post and shaking them vigorously. With the insects sufficiently enraged, the shaman holds a shield at different points on the chest, arms, back, and sometimes legs of each boy's bare body.

The boys remain still and silent. They don't flinch, whimper, or protest. Instead, they raise their arms in supplication and offer no resistance to the painful stings. To do otherwise would signal weakness and prevent them from entering manhood. Plus, it would only force them to go through the ritual again.

The boys from this tribe aren't alone in their suffering. Many indigenous Indian groups in the Amazon practice similar rites of passage, although the exact form might differ. Some, like the Sateré-Maué (who live south of the Amazon River town of Parintins), use gloves instead of shields. Others employ fire or bullet ants whose venom is even more excruciating than that of the the wasps. For many of these indigenous groups, the ant- or wasp-sting ritual is more than a rite of passage. They also use it to supply warriors with strength before battle or workers with energy before hard physical exertion, such as tree-felling.

Perhaps fifteen minutes later, the worst part ends. Having withstood the stings stoically, the boys proudly slip on elaborate feather headdresses as a sign of their new status. Again, they dance for the village, although this time their movements aren't a test of endurance but rather a display of their new standing as potential husbands, warriors, and active leaders and citizens of the community.

In early January 1998, FWS special agent Daniel LeClair in Sandusky, Ohio, scanned the report on a set of Amazonian Indian feathered artifacts discovered at Dulles International Airport's mail facility. The package, sent from Manaus, Brazil, to Jeffrey Sadofsky in South Euclid, Ohio (near Cleveland), had arrived at Dulles in late June 1997.

Contraband is often shipped through the mail. Smugglers rely on the high volume of packages to reduce the chances that their particular package will be examined.

But the shipment to Sadofsky hadn't been that lucky.

A routine inspection by a Customs official tasked with stopping illegal goods at the border led to close scrutiny of the package. Thinking it contained wildlife parts, the Customs officer called the nearest FWS wildlife inspector, Richard Potvin, to examine the contents. FWS posts just under 115 wildlife inspectors at 17 designated ports and 20 other locations[8] to process legal wildlife-related shipments and look for illegal wildlife smuggling.[9]

Potvin had recognized that the feathered artifacts in the package might contain parts from protected species and had transferred the contents to the FWS wildlife forensics lab for identification on July 23, 1997. At that time, however, the lab didn't have a forensic ornithologist on staff (one had recently left and they hadn't yet hired a new one). As a result, on September 4, 1997, the lab sent the package's twenty-eight pieces to the Smithsonian, which examined them and returned them to the lab. The lab then prepared an evaluation report based on this analysis. Meanwhile, someone from Florida asked the U.S. Postal Service about the location of the package and was told it had been detained for closer inspection.

As the officer physically closest to the package's intended recipient (Sadofsky), LeClair had been assigned to the case and now went through the evidence, including the forensic analysis from the lab. The agent lifted the crumpled newspaper from the top to see what it was all about for himself. A medicinal smell of mothballs assaulted him, and he quickly understood why: the sender had wanted to protect the fragile and perishable contents from the army of pests that might've devoured the feathered artifacts inside. With rubber-gloved hands he lifted out an elaborate but delicate feathered crown from the Kayapó Indians in Pará State in northern Brazil, including what looked like macaw tail feathers intricately woven into a stiff band that would fit an adult-sized head. He also found Wai-Wai earrings, a cheek piece, and a necklace; Kayapó belts, head adornments, and headdresses; a Kayabi necklace made with animal teeth; a Karajá apron; and other feathered handicrafts, including arm adornments. Together, the shipment was worth about $3,000.

The package had come from Manaus, a "wild west" town of almost 1.5 million people that lay in the heart of Brazil's Amazon rain forest. The Amazon is the largest rain forest in the world, comprising 2.5 million square miles across nine countries[10] with its largest portion, 60 percent, or about 1.6 million square miles, in Brazil.

Covering nearly half of Brazil, the Amazon's vast size, limited accessibility, and abundant rare and endemic species have given rise to a booming wildlife smuggling business. According to the Brazilian Network to Combat the Wild Animal Trafficking (RENCTAS), a nonprofit wildlife trade monitoring organization, Brazil's black market in wildlife is worth about a billion dollars annually and represents a sizable chunk, between 5 and 15 percent, of the world's total.[11] As one *Washington Post* reporter described it, "What Colombia is to cocaine, Brazil has become to the burgeoning illegal-animal trade."[12]

LeClair scrutinized each artifact. Beginning with European explorers' first contact with South American indigenous tribes in the 1500s, feather artwork has been what art historian Barbara Braun calls one of "the most prized Indian artifacts."[13] These ritual objects were primarily collected in ethnographic and anthropological circles as mementos during expeditions. In the mid-1930s, for example, French anthropologist Claude Lévi-Strauss undertook two voyages to Brazil (Mato Grosso in 1933–35 and Rondônia in 1938), where he collected over fifteen hundred artifacts that included many feathered works.[14] More recently (since the early 1990s), art collectors have come to value their exquisite artistry, while exhibitions at art and anthropology museums, from the Houston Museum of Natural Science, the Cantor Arts Center of Stanford University, the University Museum of Archaeology and Anthropology at the University of Pennsylvania to the Grand Palais in Paris and the Museum für Völkerkunde in Frankfurt have showcased and popularized this work.

Many of the artifacts in the package were beautiful enough to have been displayed at one of these exhibits. Some appeared well-worn while others looked new. Collectors preferred well-used older pieces, valuing them for their authenticity, but as demand for the artifacts blossomed, budding entrepreneurs capitalized on the expanding market and sought out indigenous communities to make new pieces in the traditional style. Often, these traders also "spruced up" older pieces by adding large, colorful feathers to make them more striking—and expensive.

This new industry should have provided much-needed income to impoverished communities. Instead, it often only financed the middlemen. Through the early 2000s, tourists in Brazil could readily find Indian feather art for sale in museum shops, and collectors in the United States and elsewhere could easily buy it through primitive art galleries or over the Internet.

The sharp increase in demand for feather artifacts jeopardized their source—the already vulnerable parrots, macaws, and other birds that sport the exotic plumage. While certain traditional Indian communities used to keep some types of birds in captivity as a way to retrieve their molted feathers, the practice doesn't make good economic sense: it's easier, and cheaper, to just kill them and pluck them bald, especially when a lot of feathers are needed.

Given the failure to declare the package and its Brazilian origins, LeClair suspected the artifacts might have been smuggled. He was concerned because the tropical birds that supplied the main source material were already under threat.

Birds are the animals most frequently found in Brazil's illegal trade, due to their large size and stunning diversity (the country ranks third worldwide with nearly 1,700 different bird species).[15] A good portion of illegally traded birds are for the wild bird pet trade, with about 1.5 million live birds exported each year. However, that number represents a tiny fraction of the birds actually captured because the vast majority—ten birds for every one that makes it—don't survive the trip.[16] Indeed, Brazil's illicit pet trade, combined with habitat loss, has made the world's 330 parrot species (of the family *Psittacidae*) now one of the most threatened bird families.[17]

In 1992, the United States banned the import of live wild macaws through the Wild Bird Conservation Act, and expanded the act in 1993 to include all birds on the CITES lists. The restrictions on pet macaws had largely been based on the work of American ornithologist Charles Munn, who found that only 10 to 20 percent of wild macaw pairs attempted to reproduce each year, and as few as 6 percent of chicks actually fledged.[18] The birth rates could not keep up with the high capture rates. Yet low reproduction rates and the pet trade aren't the only threat. Deforestation and hunting also affect the species.

The Wild Bird Conservation Act focuses on live birds for the pet trade and other laws, including the Migratory Bird Treaty Act (which makes it illegal to take, import, export, possess, buy, sell, or purchase any migratory bird or its feathers or other parts, nests, eggs, or products), the Endangered Species Act (which restricts take, possession, and trade in birds and their parts that are categorized as endangered or threatened), and the Eagle Protection Act (which makes it unlawful to import, export, take, sell, purchase, or barter any bald eagle or golden eagle, their parts, products, nests, or eggs, with exceptions for use by Native Americans), applied to trade in the feathers and parts from threatened and endangered birds.

According to the wildlife forensics lab's report, dated September 18, 1997, many of the artifacts destined for Sadofsky contained feathers from protected species. These included the scarlet macaw (*Ara macao*) and hyacinth macaw (*Anodorhynchus hyacinthinus*), protected under CITES Appendix I, and six species, blue-and-yellow macaw (*Ara ararauna*), red-billed toucan (*Ramphastos tucanus*), green-winged macaw (*Ara chloroptera*), yellow-crowned Amazon (*Amazona ochrocephala*), orange-winged Amazon (*Amazona amazonica*), and common rhea (*Rhea americana*), protected under CITES Appendix II. Importation of CITES-listed wildlife and their parts without proper permits violated the Lacey Act. The shipment was clearly illegal.

Yet questions remained: was this a single incident or part of a larger smuggling scheme?

LeClair, like all wildlife special agents, had a lot of leeway in deciding how to pursue the case. If he chose, he could simply issue the addressee of the package, Sadofsky, a citation and be done with it. But LeClair felt a familiar tickle of suspicion—nothing concrete, just a sixth sense that the shipment could be the tip of an iceberg. He relied on his instincts because they rarely failed him. He was a skilled officer with a keen intuition for wildlife crime. In his more than two decades in wildlife law enforcement, first as a state fish and game officer, then as regional enforcement supervisor in Iowa, and now as a special agent for FWS in the northern district of Ohio, he'd earned his reputation as an exceptional and dedicated agent. Over the years, he'd investigated everything from Great Lakes commercial fisheries involving Canadian commercial fishermen and a government-subsidized business to endangered species cases, to the smuggling of hunting trophies by Safari Club International members, to migratory bird mortalities from oil pits, to chemical poisonings, to the illegal take and sale of a trophy white-tail deer horn in interstate commerce. LeClair didn't realize it at the time but this case would become the most significant and wide-ranging of the international smuggling cases he'd worked to date.

Each new investigation energized him. A veteran law enforcement officer, LeClair had always loved nature and the outdoors. His tanned round face, stocky build, and casual dress underscored his earthy character and easy disposition. Growing up in upstate New York near Plattsburgh, he took regular outings and watched television programs like *Lassie* with his forest ranger owner and *Wild Kingdom,* which inspired him to protect the animals he cared so much about. He was the old-fashioned kind of "beat cop" who worked off his gut. If something didn't "smell" right, he dogged it until he reached the root of the crime.

LeClair's investigation would be the first time FWS had pursued such a significant investigation into artifacts containing feathers from threatened or endangered Amazon birds.

LeClair first tried to interview Sadofsky at his home on January 31, 1998. He believed Sadofsky could be the last link in a long smuggling chain, and he hoped the man would help him unearth the supplier. But during their first encounter, Sadofsky revealed little. He said he had other commitments and couldn't talk, but he let it drop that the articles in the package were supposed to have come from someone in Florida. That corresponded with the inquiries the U.S. Postal Service had initially received about the package, just after its seizure.

But Sadofsky wouldn't go further and provide the dealer's name.

Two days later, LeClair tried again. This time, the agent entered Sadofsky's house and spoke with him at greater length. Sadofsky had been collecting tribal art for twenty-five years, and two curio cabinets bursting with this primitive artwork in the living room attested to his hobby. However, Sadofsky denied any relationship to the artifacts in the package, claiming not only that he had never ordered anything from Brazil, but also that he had no relatives there, had never been to South America, and had no idea why the shipment was sent to him, except that it might be a gift from someone he didn't know. He suggested that LeClair contact the Brazilian shipper for more information.

Sadofsky also recanted his earlier mention of a supplier from Florida. When pressed, he said he couldn't remember the dealer's name and that any calls he might have made over the weekend to someone there had nothing to do with the Brazilian shipment.

LeClair thought he was lying. The backpedaling and denials merely reinforced his feeling that there was much more to the story. The agent decided to play hardball. Maybe with an indictment hanging over his head, Sadofsky would give up his supplier.

On June 10, 1998, almost a year after the initial discovery of the package at Dulles, Sadofsky and his lawyer met with LeClair and Assistant U.S. Attorney Phillip Tripi at Tripi's Cleveland office. Tripi offered to lower the felony Lacey Act charge against Sadofsky (for knowingly smuggling illegal wildlife items containing CITES-listed and endangered species into the United States without proper permits) to a misdemeanor and fine if he provided information about who arranged the import of the Brazilian Amazon Indian artifacts.

This time, Sadofsky didn't hesitate before talking. Noting that he'd dealt with the dealer only over the telephone, Sadofsky named Milan Hrabovsky (also known as Milan Harris), owner of Rain Forest Crafts in Gainesville, Florida, as the dealer of the Amazonian handicrafts.

With a name finally in hand, LeClair started his investigation in earnest. Over the next year, he researched Hrabovsky and discovered that he ran several similar businesses: Rain Forest Crafts, Rain Forest Arts, Tribal Arts, and Morpho Ventures. He also learned that the dealer had close Brazilian connections, was married to a Brazilian woman, and that his sister-in-law had sent the package to Sadofsky. Most important, LeClair uncovered how Hrabovsky operated—over the Internet and by exhibiting at craft shows around the country.

Using this information, LeClair sought approvals within FWS to launch a covert operation aimed at establishing that Hrabovsky was more than an occasional dealer but rather someone who regularly flaunted the law by importing restricted feathered artifacts.

Meanwhile, Hrabovsky remained ignorant of the pending investigation and carried on business as usual. An intelligent man who spoke four or more languages, he specialized in Native South American art and was extremely knowledgeable. He'd worked toward a Ph.D. in the subject and spent about eight years in the Amazon Basin during the mid-1970s putting together a collection for the National Museum of Japan. He didn't live lavishly but rather traveled frequently to collect specimens (he had a massive insect collection) and learn about remote societies.

Before LeClair's covert investigation started (and unbeknownst to the agent), however, Hrabovsky stumbled twice into legal hot water. In late January 1999, Brazilian authorities detained the dealer thinking he was a buyer smuggling seeds. At the same time, they seized a shipment of artifacts destined for the United States at the Eduardo Gomes Airport in Manaus that contained 784 artifacts decorated with feathers, leather, and teeth from CITES Appendix I and II species, including over 60 rattles, almost 30 purses, over 100 necklaces, and more than 130 spears, bows, and arrows. But they didn't realize its importance and relationship to Hrabovsky's illegal business. He soon traveled back to the United States, where he continued exhibiting at craft shows around the country.

On March 27, 1999, he again encountered legal trouble. This time he was at an annual spring Native American arts-and-crafts show in Collinsville, Illinois, hawking his feathered headdresses, blow guns, quivers, and necklaces when a spear with harpy eagle fletching (the feathers at the end of the spear) caught the attention of an FWS special agent.

As Hrabovsky raved to a potential client about how the six-inch smoky-brown harpy eagle feather fletching at the end of the rod invoked the animal's power, keen eyesight, and hunting prowess, FWS special agent Donnie Grace overheard and couldn't help but note the potential legal violation. He was at the show looking for breaches of the Native American Graves Protection and Repatriation Act (NAGPRA), a federal law prohibiting trafficking in Native American sacred objects and objects of cultural patrimony, and when he overheard the word "eagle," his ears perked up. Harpy eagles were protected by the Endangered Species Act, which prohibited possession of their parts (except when used by Native Americans in traditional rituals), and by CITES, which listed them under Appendix I, which banned commercial trade in their parts. Single harpy eagle feathers sold for about $40, while a spear like this one, with several plumes, went for between $70 and $90.

Grace confiscated the spear, explained the law, and issued Hrabovsky a violation notice. As the importer of the item, Hrabovsky was supposed to procure the necessary permits, but he hadn't. He admitted importing the eagle feathers into the United States from Brazil in his personal baggage and subsequently paid a $1,000 fine to dispose of the charge. Although a minor episode at the time, the incident would haunt the dealer years later when it proved that he knew that selling artifacts with feathers from protected species was against the law.

In July 1999, LeClair made his first contact with Hrabovsky through an AOL e-mail account set up expressly for this purpose. LeClair intended both to prove Hrabovsky's illegal smuggling and also reveal the extent of his market. To do that, the agent needed to uncover the kinds of species traded and the breadth of Hrabovsky's client base, since it was they who drove the trade. He would use a two-pronged approach: posing as a novice art collector, and gathering what information he could through conversations, telephone records, and tracking Hrabovsky's incoming shipments.

Through an e-mail, LeClair introduced himself to Hrabovsky, saying that someone at a flea market who had dealt with Hrabovsky in the past had suggested he contact the dealer because of their areas of mutual interest.[19]

Smugglers like Hrabovsky often use on-line auctions such as eBay and Internet websites to find their clients, and e-mail to conduct their business. Electronic communications are often more difficult to track than paper records and the old-fashioned mechanism of running classified ads in the newspaper. A month and a half later, Hrabovsky replied, asking for details about what LeClair liked.

Incorporating grammatical errors to bolster his masquerade as an "average Joe," the undercover agent responded that he wanted Amazonian craft items, such as aprons, headdresses, necklaces, masks, and armbands, and asked for brochures, an inventory of current pieces, and a price list. He also expressed interest in the history and tribal significance of the pieces to reinforce his cover as a budding amateur collector.

In his reply, Hrabovsky noted that he dealt mostly in featherwork and pointed to a well-known reference book, *Arts of the Amazon* edited by Barbara Braun, as a "catalog" that pictured many items he handled. In some sense, Hrabovsky's use of this authoritative resource legitimized his expertise and established him as a reputable dealer who traded in art rather than bric-a-brac.

In mid-November 1999, the two finally spoke on the telephone. LeClair used the personal contact as an opportunity to gather more details about Hrabovsky's operations. Hrabovsky mentioned that he maintained a sizable collection in Brazil and described his frequent trips to Native villages to buy handicrafts.

LeClair was impressed. The dealer was obviously intelligent and possessed considerable knowledge of his products.

The agent then tried to draw Hrabovsky into admitting knowledge of the law and the illegality of what he was doing. He alluded to problems with purchasing Native feathered crafts from Native American Indians, but the dealer ignored the bait. Instead, Hrabovsky simply said he'd send LeClair pictures of available items.

While this first set of photos did not contain any images of feathers from endangered birds, and therefore couldn't be used to incriminate Hrabovsky, the two continued to correspond, and in September 2000, LeClair at last received a set of digital photos with a good prospect: a huge "Upé" mask. Originally, Upé masks represented defeated enemy warriors, but more recently they signified spirits of tribespeople who'd died.[20] Made by the Tapirapé Indians—a tribe of about 200 who live at the mouth of the Tapirapé and Araguaia Rivers in north-eastern Mato Grosso (and share their 410-square-mile reservation with a group of Karajá Indians)—the giant, flat, semicircular mask was about 3½ feet wide by 2½ feet tall and was constructed with blue and yellow base feathers and long, thin scarlet accents around the face, most likely tail feathers from a scarlet macaw.

LeClair looked closely for feathers from scarlet macaws because the 12- to 15-inch-long ruby plumes were easily recognizable and came from a CITES Appendix I species, which required an import permit. LeClair wanted a "slam dunk," and the scarlet macaw feathers with their automatic felony charge would provide the simplest and most reliable path to a conviction. Proving all the elements for a conviction was hard enough without having to disprove the possibility that a feather might have come from a legally traded species. In LeClair's view, targeting parts that were readily identifiable with straightforward legal pro-

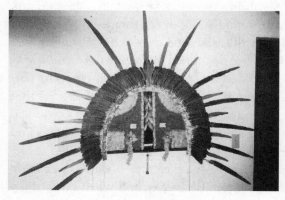

Upé mask. *(Courtesy of U.S. Fish and Wildlife Service, Office of Law Enforcement)*

tections made sense, and he would do the same for harpy eagle feathers and jaguar teeth, if and when Hrabovsky offered them.

To better make his case, however, LeClair needed two more things: hard copies of the pictures, rather than digital images, and the date the items were imported. The physical photographs could be easily linked to Hrabovsky and the artifacts because they would have his fingerprints and handwriting on them, and the import dates would help establish the illegality of the artifacts. Even if the feathers came from a protected species, if they were exported from Brazil and imported into the United States *before* the relevant laws went into effect, they would be legal. The dates would serve another purpose, too. Knowing the span of time would make it easier to check U.S. Customs and import records for the required permits.

A week later, LeClair made his first purchase: the Upé mask, with what he assumed were scarlet macaw feathers, for $1,100, and an elaborate blue "Mendko" crown with blue, yellow, red, and green feathers for $450. He didn't really need the crown, but he wanted to make a splash with this costly acquisition to solidify his cover as a serious collector.

The ploy worked. Over the next three years, LeClair and Hrabovsky maintained a regular relationship that would involve multiple purchases.

Before he proceeded further, LeClair first needed to establish that the items he'd just bought did, in fact, contain feathers from protected birds. The species identification would establish the regulations that applied and confirm violation of the law. LeClair repacked the items and sent them to the FWS wildlife forensics lab, where Pepper Trail, the newly hired forensic ornithologist, analyzed them.

Trail positively determined that the Upé mask contained feathers from scarlet macaws, a CITES Appendix I species whose trade was banned except when accompanied by special import and export permits, and from blue-and-yellow macaws, an Appendix II species that required export permits, while the blue "Mendko" crown contained feathers from two Appendix II species—blue-and-yellow macaws and red-and-green macaws.

While the species were protected, the illegality of the importation depended on when CITES had listed the species and when Hrabovsky had brought the artifacts into the United States. CITES had listed the entire macaw family in Appendix II on June 6, 1981, and the scarlet macaw individually as an Appendix I species on August 1, 1985. Given that Hrabovsky said he'd imported the items from South America about ten years earlier, in the late 1980s or early 1990s, the restrictions did apply. The "Upé" mask, with its scarlet macaw feathers, would have needed both a Brazilian CITES export permit and a U.S. CITES import permit, and the blue "Mendko" would have required a CITES export permit from Brazil.

LeClair contacted Brazilian authorities to clarify the national requirements on the export side. In a January 2001 fax, Brazil's environment protection agency, the Institute for the Environment and Renewable Natural Resources (Instituto Brasileiro do Meio Ambiente e dos Recursos Naturais Renováveis, or IBAMA), told LeClair that, as of July 7, 1998, it allowed exportation of Indian artifacts made with wildlife parts only between "official" institutions for educational, cultural, and scientific purposes and only with permits from *both* IBAMA and the government agency tasked with defending the interests and rights of Brazil's Indians: the National Indigenous Foundation (Fundação National do Índio, or FUNAI).[21]

As an individual without institutional ties, IBAMA continued, Hrabovsky couldn't even hope to receive the necessary documentation. Indeed, Brazilian authorities confirmed that Hrabovsky never obtained either the FUNAI or IBAMA permits required to export feathered Indian artifacts between educational, cultural, or scientific institutions or the necessary IBAMA permits for transporting artifacts containing CITES Appendix II–listed species.[22]

LeClair checked the U.S. side for permits for the artifacts.

They had none.

In addition, both pieces should have been declared at the U.S. border and thus been subject to FWS wildlife inspection and clearance regulations at their port of entry.

That hadn't happened.

It was a clear case of smuggling.

With a successful first "buy" under his belt, LeClair asked Hrabovsky for more pieces, ostensibly to build his collection. In reality, the agent wanted to show the full extent of Hrabovsky's criminal activities, and for that he needed more than a single purchase. Otherwise, it would be a simple buy-and-bust and a relatively minor misdemeanor.

Over the next year and a half, Hrabovsky periodically sent LeClair photos of new items, with LeClair purchasing those containing what appeared to be the distinctive long red plumes of the scarlet macaw or the sturdy dark-striped brown feathers of harpy eagles. From February 2001 to June 2002, LeClair acquired nine additional pieces for a total of $6,925. These were a Zoro crown (for $700), Saripe wasp ant glove ($750), Hixkaryana hair tube ($525), Rikbatsa crown ($650), Rikbatsa armbands ($550), Kamayura bow mask ($1,300), Arreto headdress ($650), Latiniri headdress ($900), and Rueimon flute headdress ($900). As LeClair acquired each piece, he sent it to the lab for analysis. While the lab had been unable to confirm that the artifacts contained harpy eagle feathers, the accumulated results had consistently found other protected species such as scarlet macaws, and built a broader and broader case against Hrabovsky and established him as a significant smuggler of illegal Brazilian Amazon Indian artifacts.

Yet LeClair also needed to show he wasn't Hrabovsky's only buyer. The agent knew from their conversations and communications that Hrabovsky was dealing in other places, which allowed the agent to subpoena his telephone records. The records confirmed that the dealer was traveling around the country to sell merchandise at various craft shows.

The records also revealed a number of frequently called phone numbers both in the United States, presumably those of buyers, and twenty to thirty in Brazil, most likely those of suppliers. With evidence of regular contact with Brazil, LeClair decided to track Hrabovsky's imports. He would cover all his bases. In March 2001, he requested "mail covers" that required the postal service to notify him whenever Hrabovsky received a package from Brazil.[23]

Mail covers are a service offered by the U.S. Postal Service to help with certain types of felony investigations. The process is similar to that for a search warrant. For notification for longer than sixty days, law enforcement agents must go through a postal attorney and justify the need to know about a suspect's mail and how it will help establish the commission of a crime. However, mail covers have significant limits. They only allow inspection of the outside of the package or letter. They do not authorize opening it to examine the contents. Their usefulness to LeClair would be for ascertaining the volume of material sent to Hrabovsky and identifying senders and country of origin. That information would confirm that Hrabovsky's merchandise came from Brazil and also help establish probable cause for a search warrant for future packages.

On November 19, 2001, LeClair's mail covers paid off. Until then, he hadn't received notifications of packages, perhaps because he hadn't specified the proper addresses. However, on this day he received warnings about two express mail parcels for Hrabovsky.

The agent desperately wanted to look inside. If the packages contained feathered artifacts, as he suspected, it would prove Hrabovsky imported the artifacts directly from Brazil. That would be a key step toward proving a crime because of the legal requirement for import permits.

However, the options for a covert examination were limited. The mail cover forbade him from opening the parcel, and a search warrant would be hard to get because it required probable cause, something he couldn't yet show. That left one alternative: a voluntary inspection.

But how could LeClair obtain Hrabovsky's permission?

Together with two postal inspectors, LeClair devised a ruse. A few days later, when Hrabovsky entered the University Station post office in Gainesville to pick up the two packages, the inspectors explained that, because of the recent September 11 terrorist attacks and anthrax threats, they wanted to inspect the parcels, especially since they came from a foreign address and the packaging was torn.

Hrabovsky agreed; the request seemed logical.

The two U.S. postal inspectors, Jim Podolak and Nina Schwartz, along with the local FWS special agent Andrew Aloise, who posed as a third inspector, described the procedure and had Hrabovsky sign a "Consent to Search" form that noted the voluntary nature of the search and the lack of a warrant.

With the legalities out of the way, Hrabovsky unwrapped the first package while the inspectors videotaped its contents: reed crafts, a bowl loaded with hundreds of loose, brightly colored parrot feathers, three packages of large tail feathers, and some primary feathers that appeared to be from some type of raptor. The dealer then opened the smaller package, containing ten multicolored feathered fans.

While the federal agents filmed the fans, they asked the dealer what he planned to do with items. Hrabovsky didn't want to talk. He simply said he'd imported the articles from Brazil and refused to admit that he intended to sell them.

Despite Hrabovsky's reticence to divulge the nature of his commercial activities, the agents had what they needed: evidence that the packages contained undeclared feathered artifacts without the appropriate permits. That would establish probable cause and make it easy to obtain a search warrant the next time.

Eight months later, in July 2002, that's exactly what they did. The postal service notified LeClair and Aloise of another Global Express Mail Package for Hrabovsky at the same Gainesville post office, and this time they got a warrant. November's voluntary inspection had made it a pro forma process because they could now prove that the dealer imported artifacts from Brazil without permits or declaration of the wildlife parts required by law.

Again, the parcel for Hrabovsky contained several elaborate feathered headdresses and fans, which Aloise photographed and videotaped. He then cut sixteen pieces off the feathers, in places where they wouldn't be missed, for evaluation by the lab. Finished with his collection of evidence, he resealed the package and put it back into the mail stream for delivery.

Hrabovsky would be none the wiser.

The next month, August 2002, LeClair examined a photograph Hrabovsky had sent of his latest offering. This one pictured a circular ring of hundreds of feathers, with layers of small black and red ones near the center giving way to soft yellow, blue-tipped plumes that were set off by the dark dramatically striped ones behind them. At the bottom in the middle, a bunch of black feathers with shocking white tips would hang down the wearer's back.

Hrabovsky had scrawled a brief explanation on the back:

RIKBATSA SHAMAN'S CROWN
$1000
THIS IS A CEREMONIAL
CROWN WITH HARPY EAGLE
FEATHERS ON TOP

I PREFER NOT TO DISCUSS
IT OVER THE INTERNET TOO
MUCH—I DO NOT TRUST IT
COMPLETELY.
IT IS ABOUT 30 YEARS OLD,
AND WAS BROUGHT HERE ABOUT
ONE YEAR AGO.
YOU CAN E MAIL ME IF YOU
ARE INTERESTED
THANKS.

At last Hrabovsky had written something that indicated he knew what he was doing was wrong.

Also, Hrabovsky specifically said that this piece contained harpy eagle feathers. Over the last year and a half, LeClair had bought several items that he'd thought contained harpy eagle feathers—a Hixkaryana hair tube, a Kamayura bow mask, and a Rikbatsa Indian crown. But each time the lab could not identify them as such. In fact, the lab had completely negated any chance that they even might have come from harpy eagles. Instead, for each of those pieces, it'd said that the raptor feathers were "inconsistent with harpy eagle."

LeClair still wanted to find an artifact with harpy eagle feathers to broaden the range of Appendix I species smuggled by Hrabovsky and illustrate the wide variety of birds involved. They were also important because Hrabovsky had been cited previously for illegal import of harpy eagle feathers. Therefore LeClair could prove Hrabovsky knew that what he was doing was a crime and lay the groundwork for a more serious charge.

A few weeks later, LeClair received the crown and sent it to the lab for identification.

"Beautiful," he wrote Hrabovsky. "Another addition to my already impressive collection."

CHAPTER EIGHT

Fly-by-Night Evidence

Pepper Trail, the lab's forensic ornithologist, swung his stool toward his feather-filled worktable and scanned the evidence submittal forms. He'd received a number of items from LeClair in previous shipments, but this time LeClair had sent just one item: a Rikbatsa shaman's crown.

As a young boy growing up near the Finger Lakes in upstate New York, Trail could never fully satisfy his curiosity about nature. His interest deepened during a family trip to Mexico at the age of twelve, which also sparked an ardor for travel and love of the tropics that would carry on through his professional career. Following receipt of a B.A. from Cornell University and an M.S. from the University of California–Davis, he returned to Cornell for a Ph.D. in ornithology, where his passion led him to South America for doctoral research that was later featured in *National Geographic*. After working at the Smithsonian Tropical Research Institute, the California Academy of Sciences, and as the senior wildlife biologist for the American Samoan government, he arrived at the lab in 1998. Trail's museum skills and ornithological field experience were a perfect fit for the lab's needs. He joined first on a contract basis and then was hired full-time in 1999 as a forensic ornithologist charged with identifying feathers and other bird parts, such as bones, submitted in wildlife crime investigations.

Despite his extensive training as a biologist and ornithologist, Trail had much to master on the job. In his previous work as a field biologist and later as a leader of bird-watching natural history tours (something he still did), Trail had numerous clues, such as its size, shape, and plumage pattern, to identify a bird's species. Characteristics such as the bird's geographical location, habitat, vocalizations, flight pattern, diet, and other behavior also served as pointers. At the lab, however, he usually had just a fragment to go on—often only an isolated feather.

His job ran the gamut from identifying the kinds of birds killed by poisoning from open oil pits to identifying the species of feathers or bird parts used in art, fashion, and other decoration. While the lab doesn't accept live animals, occasionally he's been asked to identify birds smuggled live in PVC tubes hidden in people's luggage (which he's done through videos or by going on-site) or determine the species of birds inside eggs that were concealed in specially made incubation vests and then smashed by the smuggler when detected at the border. While Trail's dark, hippie-ish beard made him appear as though he'd be more comfortable hiking through the rain forest than working in the lab's exacting environment, he was equally at home, and adept, in both.

The 20X24-inch circular crown covered almost his entire workspace. Well-versed in Amazonian ecology, biology, and culture, he admired its beauty and intricate design. Over one hundred feathers of varying lengths and colors had been woven into a basketry "base," giving the crown its circular shape. Different colors and sizes of feathers formed concentric rings, first black, then red, then yellow, then larger yellow feathers with blue tips, and finally an outermost ring of large, strikingly barred gray, brown, and black feathers. In the middle of the circular base, where the ends tied together, a number of large black feathers with white tips provided a dramatic asymmetrical element.

Trail was to identify all wildlife parts.

Species identification makes up a good portion, probably 75 percent, of the lab's work. For the morphology division, that number is closer to 99 percent. In all crime investigations, identifying the victim is a vital first step. In wildlife crime investigations, however, it is essential to establish the existence of a crime because some species are protected and others are not. The lab's morphologists routinely identify evidence by answering questions such as: Is this ivory carving made from warthog or elephant? Are these feathers from turkey or eagle? Is the wool shawl from cashmere goats or rare Tibetan antelope? In each instance, the second of the examples would prove an illicit activity while the first would not because trade in the species is legally allowed.

The morphology unit encompasses three taxonomically distinct areas of science: herpetology, the study of reptiles and amphibians; ornithology, the study of birds; and mammalogy, the study of mammals.

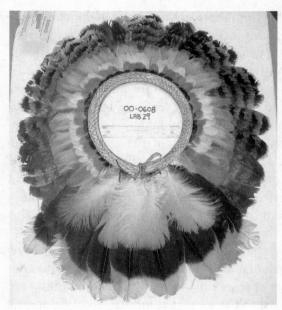

Rikbatsa shaman's crown.
(Courtesy of U.S. Fish and Wildlife Service Forensics Laboratory)

Its scientists use classic comparative anatomy techniques and also rely on their knowledge of evolution, taxonomy, geography, and animal function to identify species from their parts or remains. In addition, the lab's herpetologists, ornithologists, and mammalogists develop specialized knowledge about specific parts, such as leathers for reptiles, feathers for birds, and hair, teeth, and claws for mammals.

At first glance, the morphology department's species identifications may seem easier than those of other departments because it tends to receive evidence in somewhat recognizable forms: teeth, claws, hide, feathers, or fur. Although those items are usually part of an object, such as a purse, necklace, or piece of art, at least the morphologists can distinguish what they are. Yet knowing what an item *is* and knowing what species of animal it came from are two very different conclusions—and the latter is far from straightforward.

Identification of a species using feathers alone is complicated. To make a forensic identification, Trail first needed to figure out if a feather from a particular species was unique to that species. Sometimes, feathers from one part of the bird, such as the tail or wing, have diagnostic characteristics, while those from another part, such as the breast, would not be distinguishable from those of other birds in the same family. There are many such examples. Red-tailed and rough-legged hawks can usually be told apart by wing feathers, and always by tail feathers, but generally cannot be distinguished with certainty based on body feathers. Scarlet and red-and-green macaws are another such pair; sometimes these can be told apart by body feathers, but that depends on their exact location on the body. Trail would also need to account for variation between males and females of the same species and between stages in the bird's life. Because most birds possess about five thousand feathers, a monumental task lay ahead of the scientist.

Examining the sizes, patterns, colorations, and textures of the feathers on the crown, Trail had some good ideas of where to start. The innermost ring of tiny, half-inch black feathers had a steely blue iridescence, fine fringe, and fan-shaped profile. That suggested they were body feathers from the back of a large-bodied bird such as a curassow. While numerous curassow species exist in South America, only two genera,[1] *Pauxi* and *Mitu,* exhibit this exact combination of color and shape. From a probability standpoint, however, it was unlikely they came from the *Pauxi* group because that genus included only two very localized and rare species, *Pauxi pauxi,* the northern helmeted curassow, which lived solely in Venezuela and Colombia, and *Pauxi unicornis,* the southern helmeted curassow, found only in the eastern foothills of the Andes in Peru and Bolivia. Similarly, it was doubtful they came from three of the four species within the genus *Mitu*: *Mitu mitu,* the Alagoas curassow found only in Brazil's Atlantic coastal forest and possibly extinct in the wild; *Mitu tomentosa,* a crestless curassow from Colombia and Venezuela; and *Mitu salvini* or Salvin's curassow of Colombia, Ecuador, and Peru. That left *Mitu tuberosa,* a razor-billed curassow common throughout much of Amazonia.

While the lab's scientists try to narrow the range of options to the lowest and most specific category they can, sometimes the close relationship and resemblance between species in the same genus make it impossible to distinguish them based on partial remains, such as isolated feathers. When that happens, the scientists bring their identification to the lowest level they can, preferably to the species level but sometimes only to the genus or family. The shiny, scalloped black body feathers from each of the four species had no unique characteristics. Therefore, Trail officially left his identification at the more general, genus level and concluded that they could be either *Pauxi* or *Mitu.*

Trail hypothesized that the second inner ring of small, 1- to 1½-inch vivid red feathers served as body feathers for either the red-and-green macaw or the scarlet macaw. Body feathers provide insulation, a smooth aerodynamic silhouette, and either camouflage or signal the species or gender. Trail based his guesses on his knowledge of these birds' appearance and habits.

From their distinctive texture, Trail recognized the next layer of 2-inch light yellow feathers as underwing coverts. Because this type of feather is positioned beneath the wing at its base, they are protected from the elements and have a flimsy quality and slightly shiny surface. Given their coloration, Trail figured they once belonged to a blue-and-yellow macaw.

The penultimate, fourth, ring of larger, 2- to 3-inch yellow feathers with bluish tips also came from a scarlet macaw, Trail believed, but these were upperwing coverts. Upperwing coverts are also positioned at the base of wings but on the exterior to protect the important flight feathers. Because they're constantly exposed to sun, rain, and wind, they're strong, sturdy feathers. On the scarlet macaw, the upperwing coverts form a striking yellow "shoulder patch" that is one of the bird's most unique features. No other bird with similar-sized contour feathers has this same, distinctive pattern.

Trail turned to the 12-inch-long white-tipped black feathers at the bottom of the crown that served as a stunning accent. Given their large size, he figured they had to be from either game birds, such as curassows or turkeys, or raptors, such as eagles or hawks. From their broad flat outlines and lack of aerodynamic shape, Trail knew these were tail feathers. Tail feathers provide lift and increase maneuverability and, like wing feathers, their shape varies in a predictable way according to their position on the tail. Central tail feathers have symmetrical vanes (that is, the cohesive sheets of soft feather material) on either side of the shaft to increase the tail's surface area and supply more lift. Outer tail feathers possess progressively narrower outside vane edges to stiffen the plume so that it can better withstand the greater air resistance of those positions. From their hefty size, black color, and broad white tips, Trail could tell at once that these, too, must have come from either *Mitu* or *Pauxi*, just like the small black body feathers. Yet this time he had more to go on than probabilities and geography. As is often the case with bigger feathers, these tail feathers exhibited unique characteristics that let him distinguish between species. Specifically, the white tips ruled out two of the four *Mitu* species, *Mitu mitu* and *Mitu tomentosa*, whose tail feathers have brown tips. Moreover, the tail feathers of *Pauxi* and of Salvin's curassow always have a greenish sheen, which these didn't. Putting together all these characteristics, Trail knew these feathers could only have come from the relatively widespread razor-billed curassow (*Mitu tuberosa*).

Last, Trail examined the outer ring of spectacular 5- to 6-inch barred and mottled feathers around the outside of the crown. Their color fluctuated from gray to brown to black, with the brightness of the stripes varying in intensity. A number of birds, including raptors, game birds, and owls, have barring (stripes). Trail immediately eliminated owls because these didn't have the fuzzy texture that deadens an owl's sound during flight. He also ruled out game birds because the large size, gray tones, and details of the patterning on these feathers wasn't right.

That left raptors, which often have the complex mottled patterns like these for better camouflage.

With high-powered magnifying visors, Trail examined the central spines, or shafts, of the feathers for confirmation. No question. The dark, solid spines indicated that the feathers came from a bird of prey. On a game bird, the shafts would have displayed fine parallel lines running lengthwise *inside* the shaft.

He turned the artifact over to inspect the underside of the shaft. Again, he found characteristics of raptors—distinctive V-shaped grooves, as if they'd been cut with a knife—rather than those of game birds (U-shaped ones, as if they were scooped with a spoon). These were *definitely* from a bird of prey.

To narrow it further, Trail assessed the position of the feather on the bird's body. These weren't stiff, strong, or big enough to be flight feathers from either the wing or tail. They also weren't the right shape. Their symmetry pointed to body (also called contour) feathers, which, as Trail explained, "experience life the same on both sides."[2] The scientist figured these were upperwing coverts. That knowledge, combined with what was a huge size for a contour feather, narrowed the range of possible raptors to the largest of all: eagles. Contour feathers from hawks and other raptors are smaller.

But which eagle species?

Around the world, over fifty eagle species exist, but the circumstances of this case allowed Trail to restrict his options geographically. He focused on the two largest Amazon-based species: harpy and crested eagles.

From his forensic experience and extensive field research in the region, Trail's gut told him these were harpy eagle feathers. Harpy eagles have a fairly distinct plumage pattern—dark brown with blacker barring and complex mottling—that seemed to match these feathers.

Yet Trail couldn't rely on only a cursory visual exam. Even when the lab's scientists have excellent ideas of the species of an animal part or product, they must always go a step further and verify their hypotheses against known examples. As Espinoza did with bear bile, Trail needed to confirm his initial assumptions by comparing the evidence feathers to reference samples or standards. That would complete his analysis and make it defensible in court.

The collection of known specimens is central to the lab's work. Without it, the lab couldn't do its job because it wouldn't be able to make a definitive evaluation. The lab maintains a significant reference collection for species of interest to law enforcement. Unfortunately, it had no harpy eagle or crested eagle standards, which meant Trail could not make detailed comparisons between the two. While numerous detailed reference images confirmed Trail's expert assessment, they weren't enough. Some crested eagles shared the basic plumage pattern, and without a good specimen to act as a standard, Trail couldn't be certain of his conclusion beyond a reasonable doubt. As a result, he left his identification at what he could verify with absolute certainty: the half-foot-long barred feathers came from *either* crested or harpy eagles.

To confirm the other feather identifications, Trail gathered the necessary reference samples from the room next to his lab. The room housed a series of plain beige cabinets containing the morphology unit's standards, including a sizable collection of seven thousand bird specimens that represented about a thousand separate species, or 10 percent of the world's bird species.[3]

The lab's specimen collection targets representative samples of species of interest, or the most frequent victims of crimes. Parts of the collection, such as prepared skins, skulls, and skeletons, are similar to those found at natural history museums. Other parts, however, such as hair, loose feathers, reptile leather, or finished products, are more specialized and tailored to the exacting needs of wildlife forensics.

Unlike the massive collections maintained by major institutions such as the Smithsonian Institution, Chicago's Field Museum of Natural History, and New York's American Museum of Natural History, the lab's reference standards are used primarily for identification rather than for documenting the complete range of variation within a species. Generally, the lab doesn't need as wide-ranging a collection because, in most cases, a few specimens suffice to document a species' basic plumage types for identification purposes.

Trail slid out a shallow four-foot-long drawer filled with over a dozen large stuffed birds. Their blank cotton eyes stared up at him as he carefully picked up the blue-and-yellow, red-and-green, and scarlet macaws.

Back at his desk, Trail scrutinized the preserved birds. The crown's

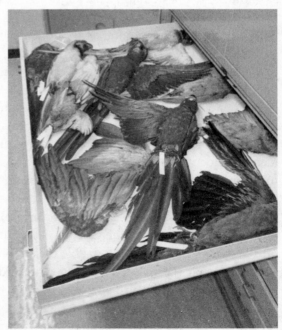

Macaw reference samples.
(Courtesy of Laurel A. Neme)

light yellow underwing coverts exhibited the same shade of pale yellow with an occasional spot of blue-gray at the tip as the lab's blue-and-yellow macaw standard.

The red-and-green and scarlet macaws appeared remarkably similar at first glance. The chests of both were bright red, covered with small feathers that were indistinguishable in size and shape. On closer inspection, however, Trail noticed extremely subtle differences in hue: the red-and-green macaw body feathers were a slightly dusky shade of red while those of the scarlet macaw were a light, pure red with hints of yellow at the feather's base.

He placed the crown feathers side-by-side with the samples and the difference in tint compared with the red-and-green macaw was obvious. But he still had to be 100 percent certain that they were from a scarlet macaw.

With forceps, he moved some of the crown's feathers aside for a better look at their bases. Near where the small red feathers attached to the crown he saw light red with yellow and compared them with the scarlet macaw feathers. They matched perfectly.

He did the same with the blue-tipped yellow feathers.

No question: both came from scarlet macaws.

Special Agent LeClair reviewed Trail's September 2002 forensic report on the Rikbatsa shaman's crown. The scientist had definitively determined that it contained feathers from scarlet macaws (*Ara macao*), blue-and-yellow macaws (*Ara ararauna*), razor-billed curassows (*Mitu tuberosa*), and either harpy or crested eagles.

The laws applying to each of these birds were as complex as those applied to black bears. The razor-billed curassow wasn't protected, so LeClair ignored that identification for purposes of building his case. While the harpy eagle was protected under CITES Appendix I (listed July 1, 1975) and the Endangered Species Act, the less-threatened crested eagle fell under CITES Appendix II (listed on June 28, 1979). However, the lack of a positive identification of harpy eagle from the lab, combined with the lesser protections for the alternative—crested eagles—prevented these feathers from supplying the conclusive "slam dunk" LeClair wanted for his case. To get it, the agent shipped the harpy eagle feathers in the crown to an FWS wildlife inspector in Chicago, who walked them over to the Field Museum of Natural History. There, a scientist used the museum's extensive reference collection and positively identified the feathers as harpy eagle.

LeClair also focused on the lab's definitive scarlet macaw identifications. Hrabovsky had said he'd imported the item from Brazil about a year earlier in 2001, well after the 1985 CITES Appendix I listing for the species. That meant the Rikbatsa shaman's crown, with its scarlet macaw feathers, would have needed both a Brazilian CITES export permit and a U.S. CITES import permit. Yet to prove the crime, LeClair first had to do what he'd done for every piece he'd bought: verify that the crown had no permits.

To hide his businesses, Hrabovsky had played a shell game and employed multiple names and addresses. If a permit had been issued for the handicraft under an assumed name and LeClair didn't catch it, the entire case would be called into question. To avoid mistakes arising from the subterfuge, LeClair collected the names of all Hrabovsky's aliases and associates, over a dozen in total, and checked the records for each of the possibilities.

Nothing.

As with all the other artifacts, nobody had asked about or received a permit for the Rikbatsa shaman's crown.

The case against Hrabovsky was growing stronger.

On October 23, 2002, LeClair closed the covert part of the operation. When the investigation started three and a half years earlier, Hrabovsky was married, lived at a single address, and ran his businesses from his home. But his personal circumstances had changed—he and his wife had divorced and he now bunked with a couple of friends, changing addresses frequently and sometimes living out of his vans—he had little to tie him down, and LeClair suspected he was ready to bolt. Recently, he had heard rumblings that the dealer was heading to Asia. LeClair had enough evidence against the dealer, and if he didn't make an arrest soon, he might lose his quarry. Besides, LeClair had fulfilled his goal of showing the range of Hrabovsky's dealings.

With the investigation complete and the lab's evidence providing probable cause, LeClair obtained search warrants for two apartments in Gainesville, a storage unit, and two vans, as well as an arrest warrant for the dealer himself. The agent hoped to find an inventory of additional artifacts and business records that would further prove the extent of his smuggling.

At dawn on October 23, 2002, five teams composed of forty FWS and state wildlife enforcement officers, U.S. Immigration and Customs officials, and local police began their search of Hrabovsky's properties. The two apartments yielded two computers, a scanner, business records, photographs, telephone records, correspondence, and passports, as well as artifacts, macaw feathers, and bird bones. At one of the residences, agents also found a large envelope addressed to Hrabovsky dated March 30, 1998, from the FWS Office of Management Authority that contained the 1994 and 1996 CITES lists and regulations, with pencil and ink markings on the import and export regulations. These documents would offer invaluable help in showing Hrabovsky knew his actions were criminal.

From the van parked outside the first apartment, agents confiscated a package of photographs, including shots of a Latirina headdress, Rueimon flute headdress, and toucan headdress; a Bororo shaman's necklace; a small notebook with words written in Portuguese followed by an English translation; a sheet listing the names of birds with scientific names; and a memo from a known client of Rain Forest Crafts regarding his account balance. In addition, they seized two large garbage bags full of numerous packages of individual feathers, including those of the blue-headed parrot and the blue-and-yellow macaw, and three tribal art craft items composed of feather and bone, including two with six to twelve clusters composed of feathers from the harpy eagle and the scarlet macaw as well as from the CITES Appendix II–listed laughing falcon (*Herpetotheres cachinnans,* also referred to as the snake hawk) and mealy parrot (*Amazona farinosa*), among others.

The storage unit, too, generated a heap of evidence. Inside they found photographs, an address book, credit card slips for one of Hrabovsky's businesses, Morpho Ventures, as well as feathered handicrafts, loose feathers, and animal teeth. The artifacts varied and included several spears with unidentified feather fletching, costumes with semiplumes from curassows, crowns with scarlet macaw feathers, beaded necklaces with skin patches from the CITES Appendix II–listed channel-billed toucans (*Ramphastos vitellinus*) and others with spangled cotinga (*Cotinga cayana*) feathers, and a necklace with 109 monkey teeth (including some from a kind of capuchin monkey from the *Cebus* genus, many of which are listed in CITES Appendix II) and scarlet macaw feathers. While the eighty-four-square-foot unit was small, about the size of a small office work space, its air-conditioning provided the perfect climate control to prevent the artifacts from deteriorating.

The searches of the properties uncovered a wealth of evidence and over two dozen additional artifacts. Yet they failed to locate the primary target: Hrabovsky.

By now, LeClair knew Hrabovsky's patterns, and on a hunch he had stationed two agents at the post office. The midmorning sun cast a long shadow as Hrabovsky drove his battered blue van into the University Station post office parking lot. Next to him, between the seats, was the package containing his latest shipment for LeClair, an especially rare piece, a Bororo shaman's necklace. This was the first occasion on which Hrabovsky had sold LeClair an item containing jaguar teeth.

Jaguars are protected under Appendix I of CITES and LeClair had, of course, jumped at the chance to buy it. Jaguars are among the animals given CITES's highest level of protection, and with the Bororo shaman's necklace, LeClair could prove that Hrabovsky's dealings went far beyond birds.

With little fanfare, federal agents arrested Hrabovsky and seized the van. The vehicle contained a jumble of clothes, sleeping mats, and cooking utensils, reinforcing the impression that this battered vehicle was Hrabovsky's home, but it also contained a mother lode of evidence, including a pocket telephone/address book with listings of known customers and foreign suppliers; a box filled with files of some of Rain Forest Craft's most frequent customers, with each file identifying the customer, his or her contact information, purchases made, copies of color photographs sent, invoices, and annotations reflecting the conversations about the item and quoted cost; a purple photo album showing tribal art items for sale; a red file folder with pages listing tribal art items, suppliers, and costs (most written in Portuguese but some in English); a black folder containing business cards of some of the local aviaries in Florida, Georgia, and North Carolina that were apparently selling feathers to Hrabovsky so he could make, repair, and spruce up his merchandise; another box of files containing names, addresses, telephone numbers, invoices, and correspondence (mostly written in Portuguese) that referenced some of Hrabovsky's Brazilian suppliers; as well as the parcel for LeClair containing the Bororo shaman's necklace.

Yet that wasn't all. In addition to material from the searches, during the same period LeClair received notification about three separate express mail shipments mailed from Brazil to Hrabovsky's post office boxes, which the agent also searched. The sizable 2X1½X1-foot packages contained more of the dealer's inventory, sixty-two additional items in all. These included several bone whistles made from the ulna of unidentified birds; a wooden club with down feathers from either the harpy or crested eagle; bead necklaces, bracelets, and belts with scarlet macaw body feathers; crowns with scarlet macaw feathers; purses; ten monkey teeth necklaces; and loose feathers from harpy eagles, macaws, and other birds.

This multitude of evidence appeared to clinch the case against Hrabovsky. But the work couldn't stop there. Over the coming months, LeClair would sift through the records and follow up on every lead. That included shipping the eighty-eight additional artifacts (many with parts from multiple species) to the lab for identification.

In December 2002, Pepper Trail removed the foam wrapping that had been shrouding the Bororo shaman's necklace when it was recovered from Hrabovsky's vehicle at the post office. The necklace's highlight was the single 4X2-inch pendant, about the size of a deck of playing cards, that had been fashioned from a dark brown moldable amalgam, perhaps glue, dirt, and wood pulp mixed together and then baked until hard. A skin patch covered with 1- to 1½-inch-long sunset-hued feathers wrapped around the waxy resin while four massive fangs protruded from the bottom and signaled the wearer's power.

Lifting the necklace up by its foot-long beaded string, the scientist admired the rosettes of multicolored feathers dangling from its cord. Analyzing their color, shape, size, and texture, Trail determined that the feathers of both scarlet and red-and-green macaws were represented. The clump of yellow, orange, and red feathers on the boxlike pendant clearly came from a toucan. While most body feathers resemble a leaf, with an oval shape and definite edge, the individual barbs of toucan feathers do not interlock to form a closed outline, giving them a distinctive "hairy" appearance.

All toucans are predominantly black, with color either at their throat or tail. The colors of the throat patch vary by species, with two, namely the red-breasted toucan and the channel-billed toucan, possessing the same orange-yellow and red pattern of the feathers in this artifact. However, not having the appropriate reference standard, Trail couldn't go any further and left his evaluation there.

For analysis of the teeth hanging from the pendant, Trail turned the necklace over to Margaret "Cookie" Sims, one of the lab's two mammalogists. Sims first joined the lab as a volunteer when she was an undergraduate biology student at Southern Oregon State College and was hired as a full-time forensic specialist in 1997. She soon became an expert on ivory as her supervisor and head of the morphology section, Bonnie Yates, the senior mammalogist, consistently assigned her teeth-related casework as a way to more easily divide up the workload.

The four 2-inch-long teeth each curved outward from the center of the pendant, with two pointing right and two left. The entire structure of each tooth—root, cingulum (the junction near the gum line where the enamel stops and the root begins), and enamel—was visible. That would help with identification.

Sims recognized the shape of the four teeth as canines. Technically, the word "canine" refers to the tooth position in an animal's mouth, but carnivores' canines differ greatly from herbivores' in shape. The conical, spearlike shape of these teeth told Sims they had to come from a carnivore.

The shape of mammal teeth varies by function and position. The flatter molars of herbivores, for example, are used for grinding while their more rounded incisors help with snipping. In contrast, carnivores' "mountainlike" points, called cusps, on their molars and premolars help with crushing, shearing, and directing food while their pointy incisors are excellent for gripping and nipping.

Seeing the massive size of these canines, bigger than her thumb, Sims immediately ruled out most carnivores. They were at least twice the size of those of the canids, the dog family, including wolves, coyotes, and dogs, and far bigger than those of all the smaller carnivores, such as martens, weasels, and small cats. That meant they had come from a large carnivore, either from the cat (*Felidae*) or bear (*Ursidae*) families.

Canine teeth, especially those of bears and large cats, are prized in

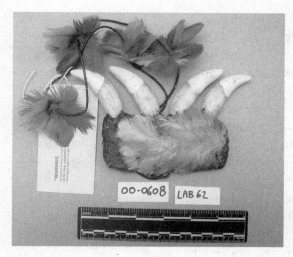

Bororo shaman's necklace.
(Courtesy of U.S. Fish and Wildlife Service Forensics Laboratory)

Native ornaments for their power and symbolism. However, when separated from the animal, they can look remarkably similar. To determine which family these came from, Sims examined the enamel-coated part of the fangs. Bears have distinctive brown rings that encircle the tooth whereas cats have pitted grooves that run from tip to base. Sometimes, these grooves appear more like cracks on both the inside and outside surfaces of the exposed part of the tooth, but Sims easily made them out on the necklace's teeth. The teeth were from a cat.

But what kind of cat? There were almost forty species.

Size alone ruled out most of them. These teeth were too small to be from a tiger or lion, the largest cats, and too big to be from smaller cats like bobcat or lynx. They had to come from one of what Sims categorized as the five medium-sized cats: mountain lions or cougars, cheetahs, leopards, snow leopards, or jaguars.

Canines within this group vary in size and shape based on skull and body size, prey type, and killing method. Cheetahs, for example, which outrun their prey, have diminutive canines to better fit inside their streamlined skulls. Canine shape, too, is specially adapted for different types of prey. The less conical-shaped canines of leopards are better suited for softer food like antelopes, while jaguars' tougher and more robust circular canines are superior for not only severing vertebrae in one bite but also stabbing open tougher fare such as turtles and reptiles.

In fact, the topic of canine function is subject to much research and debate, especially among scientists studying saber-toothed cats, who question whether that prehistoric creature's colossal canines were meant to kill prey because to do so would undoubtedly have broken the long teeth, rendering them completely useless.

Before Sims could pinpoint which of the five medium-sized cats these canines came from, she determined the position of each evidence tooth in the mouth by looking at its curvature. Two teeth were less curved and therefore came from the upper part of the jaw, while the two more curved teeth came from the lower jaw.

The orientation of the ridges on the teeth, buccal (toward the outside of the mouth) or lingual (toward the tongue), told Sims she had two from the right side of the jaw, and two from the left. The four teeth formed a set of canines, possibly from one individual cat.[4]

Knowing the position of the teeth prepared Sims for a game of matching in which she'd consult her cat skull standards. Ignoring the orderly clutter of trays of meticulously organized animal parts lining the counters and whole skeletons and stuffed animals peering down above their reference-filled perches above, she abandoned the morphology lab and marched into the next room to retrieve them.

Opening the beige metal doors of the museum cabinet, she slid open several of the foot-deep and meter-wide drawers. Each contained about two dozen skulls, a mixture of males, females, and subadults. She grabbed two or three skulls for each of the five medium-sized cat species. She needed a few representative samples of each kind to ensure that she picked up any variation that might have occurred from that animal's life experiences.

Holding the necklace up to each skull, she compared the size, curvature, grooves, and cingulum profiles—where the enamel ends and root begins—of the teeth in the necklace and the teeth of the specimen skulls.

The cheetah and cougar canines were noticeably smaller, about one-third the size; the leopard and snow leopard teeth were longer, more saberlike, and with prominent grooves. None of these were a match.

Finally, Sims compared the cingulum profile with the canines in the known jaguar skull specimens.

Jaguars are the biggest feline in the Americas, and the third largest in the world after tigers and lions. Their common name comes from the

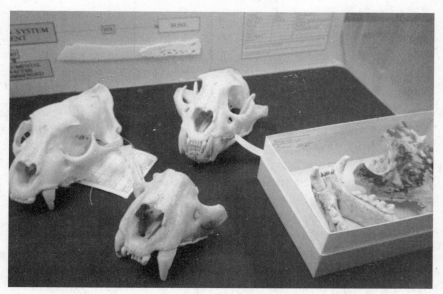

Examples of cat skull reference standards. *(Courtesy of Laurel A. Neme)*

Indian word *yaguar*, which means "he who kills with one leap,"[5] while their scientific name, *Panthera onca*, means "hunter," "hook," or "barb" and refers to their stealth and formidable claws. They look similar to leopards, except that jaguars are stockier, with shorter, more muscular limbs and smaller tails, and they have spots inside their rosettes. Their camouflage spots, which are unique to each individual; specially padded paws, which mask noise when stalking; agile tree-climbing abilities; and strong jaws and powerful killing bite combine to make them stealthy and formidable hunters.

Jaguars have long been an important symbol in indigenous American Indian culture, with many Amazonian tribes believing the reflective glow of their eyes provides a link to the spirit world.

Even though jaguars are found from Mexico across Central America and south into Paraguay and northern Argentina, there aren't many left. During the 1960s and 1970s, about 15,000 or more were killed for their dramatic fur. Now estimates of their total populations range between 10,000 and 20,000. The IUCN Red List classifies them as near threatened, and they are protected under CITES Appendix I.

Sims found that the necklace's teeth definitely came from a jaguar.

• • •

During most of December 2002, the lab's scientists evaluated the hundreds of feathers, teeth, and other parts contained in the almost one hundred items seized from Hrabovsky. With each analysis, they lengthened the list of victims. Hrabovsky's merchandise had included parts from a large variety of birds, including harpy eagles, scarlet macaws, hyacinth macaws, red-and-green macaws, blue-and-yellow macaws, green ibis, Guianan red-cotingas, spangled cotingas, Maguari storks, great egrets, orange-winged parrots, mealy parrots, bare-necked fruitcrows, laughing falcons, channel-billed toucans, aracari toucans, oropendolas, curassows, and chickens, as well as a remarkable assortment of mammals including jaguars, capuchin and other monkeys, and even armadillos.

But more important, the lab's identification of victims provided the critical link LeClair needed to make his case. It had established that Hrabovsky's activities violated the law, by proving that the animal parts came from protected species.

CHAPTER NINE

Buyer Beware

The investigation into Hrabovsky opened the floodgates to a raft of prosecutions. The wealth of evidence seized during the October 2002 searches triggered a whole new round of investigations, this time into Hrabovsky's clients and Brazilian suppliers.

During February and March 2003, LeClair and his colleagues interviewed as many of Hrabovsky's buyers as they could find. Most of the buyers identified from the business records were more than the typical middle-class citizen who bought one or two pieces at a craft fair. Rather, they were "regulars" who'd purchased a half dozen or more items worth several thousand dollars from Rain Forest Crafts over a period of several years. Sometimes, they bought their items from the dealer at his exhibitions at Native American art fairs such as the Santa Fe Ethnographic Show. Other times they shopped via electronic and regular mail. But they were all prominent, well-educated, and affluent individuals intent on building personal collections, though many also simultaneously wanted to help preserve the cultural heritage of Amazonian Indian communities.

Even without malicious intent, the result was the same. The collectors created demand for the feather art, which gave dealers such as Hrabovsky the incentive to smuggle it out of Brazil and into the United States.

LeClair's investigations initially concentrated on about twenty-five of Hrabovsky's repeat clients. The list was composed of people from all over the country, including California, Colorado, Florida, Kentucky, Maryland, Massachusetts, New Mexico, New York, North Dakota, Ohio, Utah, and Washington. Agents from every one of FWS's nine administrative law enforcement regions, except Alaska and Hawaii, helped conduct the interviews.

From these twenty-five, LeClair selected about a dozen who appeared to be Hrabovsky's largest clients and had each spent $10,000 to $20,000 on handicrafts from Rain Forest Crafts or Hrabovsky's other businesses. They included a Dickinson State University anthropology professor, owners of art galleries, and lawyers, all of whom had or should have had intimate knowledge of the law.

One of the most prominent was a former zoo director who was well-versed in issues related to endangered species. Like Hrabovsky's other buyers, Ed Maruska, who served as the director for the Cincinnati Zoo from 1968 to 2000, had a deep-rooted passion for tribal art, and spent his adult life assembling a huge personal collection of artifacts from indigenous African, Asian, and South American peoples. He'd worked tirelessly on conservation and is credited with turning the zoo into an internationally known facility with one of the top animal collections in the country. Maruska said that the record of centuries of history and beliefs contained in the artifacts, deserved equal protection. Leaving the handicrafts to rot in their original environment, where insects and humidity would have destroyed them, he argued, would have been, if not a travesty, then extremely unfortunate.

When Maruska had started doing business with Hrabovsky, he'd asked about the legality of the artifacts, and the dealer assured him he had the appropriate permits.

From 1998 until 2002, the former zoo director bought $20,000 worth of Brazilian Amazonian Indian artifacts from Hrabovsky, including high-quality items such as harpy eagle feathered arrows, a Saripe wasp ant glove like the one LeClair bought, headdresses, and necklaces. But the dealer had lied. Many of Maruska's purchases, like those of Hrabovsky's other buyers, contained parts from protected species and were therefore illegal.

Maruska, like the other clients, claimed he had practiced due diligence by asking Hrabovsky about the artifacts, and couldn't help that the dealer had deceived him. But claiming innocence is common, LeClair says.

"This is a kind of ruse that these collectors use all over the country. They place the blame elsewhere. Since someone else did the dirty work and brought the article out of Brazil, they figure they didn't commit the crime. But they still want the authentic article, so, when Hrabovsky had it, they bought it."[1]

Buyers often distance themselves from the actual point of the poaching or smuggling. That may clear their consciences but it doesn't release them from their legal obligations. Because the artifacts contained species listed under CITES Appendix I, they needed CITES export permits from Brazil and import permits from the United States, which they didn't have. The buyers should have checked—and the law agreed.

Hrabovsky's clients got off with fines and forfeiture of the artifacts. The former zoo director voluntarily surrendered his collection and later acknowledged that given his position and level of education, he should have known not to purchase items made with endangered and protected wildlife without verifying documentation or proof of their legal importation.

He wasn't alone.

Hrabovsky's other major buyers also voluntarily abandoned their collections, worth hundreds of thousands of dollars. Over a hundred artifacts were relinquished or seized.

Ten individuals were charged with misdemeanor violations. All pleaded guilty and collectively paid almost $40,000 in fines.

In the case of stolen or illegal goods, claiming ignorance rarely absolves guilt, and it never eliminates accountability. Consumers have a responsibility to know where their "stuff" comes from as well as the impact of their purchases, especially when those goods are artistic and the potential for fraud or abuse is clear, as it was with the Amazonian artifacts. When dealing with products made from rare animals, that obligation is even more essential, because it is those same buyers who fuel demand. Their desire for the goods can quickly spiral out of control and past a level where the species can safely withstand the exploitation.

As for Hrabrovsky, Assistant U.S. Attorney Gregory McMahon for the northern district of Florida in Gainesville indicted him on seventeen counts that included separate felony Lacey Act charges for each of the items purchased by LeClair, smuggling charges related to the undeclared wildlife parts in the express mail packages, and an obstruction of justice charge. They based the obstruction charge on interviews with one of Hrabovsky's clients, who'd supplied a telephone message tape in which the dealer had instructed the buyer to get rid of the artifacts. Other buyers mentioned similar actions. After Hrabovsky's October 23, 2002, arrest and subsequent release on an unsecured bond, he called several of his customers to tell them that, because of recent problems with the federal government, he wouldn't be able to conclude pending business, and said they should conceal, store, or hide their collections and not reveal his name as the seller. He also asked his customers to avoid residential phones or cell phones, because they could be traced or identified, and to use pay phones for contact instead.

With such solid evidence against Hrabovsky, a conviction looked certain.

Hrabovsky didn't have much to offer federal agents for reduced charges. They already had a lot of information about his client base and Brazilian suppliers. Nevertheless, federal authorities wanted a speedy conclusion and offered him a deal. They'd drop fourteen of the counts and agree not to indict his (now ex-) wife, who had played a major role in the business but also cared for their child, in exchange for his cooperation. Maybe they'd learn something new.

It wasn't much of deal for Hrabovsky. The federal sentencing guidelines already put his sentence in the range of between thirty-three and forty-one months of jail time. Even so, he accepted, hoping a judge might be more lenient.

Six months after LeClair's search, on March 12, 2003, Hrabovsky pleaded guilty in the U.S. District Court in Gainesville to three of the seventeen counts against him—felony Lacey Act, smuggling, and obstruction of justice.

But Hrabovsky barely cooperated. At his May 2003 debriefing by LeClair at the Federal Detention Facility in Tallahassee, Hrabovsky supplied only vague and general answers. He couldn't or wouldn't remember the names of his Brazilian suppliers or the nature of his dealings with them, and he denied receiving four parcels from Brazil in October 2002 at his Gainesville post office boxes—packages that LeClair already knew about.

Hrabovsky did say that he had a large "personal collection" of Amazonian tribal art located with relatives in the Czech Republic, but that after his arrests he'd advised his relatives to destroy the entire thing. He also stated that he wasn't selling the tribal art items that had been shipped from Brazil to relatives in the Czech Republic or to any European customers.

LeClair, however, suspected otherwise. From copies of correspondence indicating that a number of shipments with hundreds of items of Amazonian tribal art crafts were sent from Brazilian suppliers to an address in the Czech Republic, it appeared that with the help of his relatives, Hrabovsky was operating a similar business for European customers.

All in all, Hrabovsky added little new information to the investigation. Luckily, his help wasn't vital to the case. The agents already had what they needed from the seizures. From the searches, they not only had invoices and records of Hrabovsky's clients but also an address book with contact information for his suppliers and access to a multitude of faxes to Brazilian suppliers requesting merchandise and detailing purchases. That would allow Brazilian authorities to initiate a case from the supply end.

Despite the lack of cooperation from Hrabovsky, the deal ensured a swift conviction. LeClair and McMahon felt a trial would not result in any extra jail time beyond the thirty-three-month sentencing minimum and would simply be a waste of government money.

In June 2003, Senior District Court Judge Maurice Paul sentenced Hrabovsky to forty months (three years and four months) in prison— one of the longest terms ever handed down for a wildlife violation. The international scope of the case and the large scale of Hrabovsky's operation triggered tougher federal sentencing guidelines that allowed Judge Paul to confer a high penalty. That, combined with a sympathetic judge who understood the repercussions of wildlife trafficking, resulted in the tough punishment.

The judge also ordered Hrabovsky to three years' supervised probation after his release, to forfeit all his illegal wildlife items, and to repay the $9,425 FWS had spent buying the artifacts in LeClair's undercover sting.

LeClair felt satisfied with the result.

"Anytime a wildlife smuggler gets jail time," he later noted, "we've done a great job."

Typically, penalties for wildlife violations involve minimal fines, forfeiture of the illegal wildlife products, and sometimes dismissals. They rarely include significant fines or imprisonment.

By comparison, Hrabovsky received an extremely stiff sentence.

Despite his prison sentence, evidence suggests that Hrabovsky was still enthralled by the trade of artifacts and intended to carry on his smuggling businesses. In June 2004, Assistant U.S. Attorney McMahon, the prosecutor of Hrabovsky's case, learned about a storage unit that Hrabovsky had never declared.

The discovery was pure happenstance. With the rent long overdue, the storage facility owner had entered Hrabovsky's unit and found thirty boxes loaded with feathered artifacts. Not knowing what to make of them, the owner asked a local university professor for advice. That professor, in turn, remembered the federal case and called McMahon.

The implications for Hrabovsky were disastrous. The undeclared storage unit filled with Amazonian Indian handicrafts provided proof of the dealer's flagrant disregard of the terms of his plea agreement. As part of his plea bargain, he'd promised to tell authorities about and forfeit *all* of his illegal wildlife handicraft items.

He clearly hadn't.

Hrabovsky's duplicity prompted McMahon, in January 2005, to consider revoking the plea agreement and indicting Hrabovsky on *all* seventeen of the original charges. The prosecutor also indicated he'd make sure the dealer remained incarcerated for his full sentence, with no early release for good behavior.

Facing this pessimistic scenario, Hrabovsky gave up hope of any future appeal or legal salvation. In June 2005, twenty-four months into his forty-month sentence, he escaped from the Edgefield Federal Correctional Facility in Estil, South Carolina.[2] As of 2008, he remains at large.

The case against another artifacts dealer, Rosita Heredia, and her high-profile client that ran parallel to Hrabovsky's illustrates how the low priority given to wildlife trafficking stimulates the trade. It highlights, in particular, how easily buyers usually get off and how these minimal punishments spur demand.

Beginning in November 2000, FWS special agent Allen Hundley, who'd been in contact with LeClair, initiated an investigation into the Brazilian Amazon feather art collection of Lawrence Small, then secretary of the Smithsonian Institution, following its appearance in a January 2000 *Smithsonian* magazine article. The dazzling collection included a thousand headdresses, capes, masks, nosepieces, and armbands, all "festooned with feathers of every conceivable color and size, from foot-long macaw feathers to fingernail-size hummingbird feathers."[3] After seeing some of its pieces displayed at a National Geographic Society exhibit and Duke University's art museum, Small had, in 1998, bought it lock, stock, and barrel from a private dealer and Harvard-educated cultural anthropologist, Rosita Heredia, for $400,000.[4] While part of the collection, 850 pieces, had been imported by Heredia earlier (in 1984 and 1994), the remaining 150 pieces were imported once the transaction was completed.

Heredia ran an operation similar to Hrabovsky's, wherein she purchased artifacts illegally from FUNAI officials in Brazil and sold them to clients (including twenty-three items to a leading art collector and board member of the Smithsonian's Hirshhorn Museum and Sculpture Garden for $39,000 and sixteen items to an art gallery owner in New York for $31,000) in the United States.

Noticing what looked like distinctive parts from protected species such as scarlet macaws in the magazine photographs, Special Agent Hundley questioned the legality of Small's collection. During the ensuing investigation, Small, like Hrabovsky's clients, said Heredia had claimed to have the necessary permits and that he had "no knowledge that any species in the collection is listed under the Endangered Species Act."[5] As the head of one of the world's largest museums, Small probably should have known better, even though his attorney said that because portions of the collection had been on public display, Small had assumed the entire collection was legal.[6]

Trail and the other scientists at the FWS wildlife forensics lab analyzed Small's collection and found that 206 items contained feathers, teeth, and other parts from species including harpy eagle, scarlet macaw, hyacinth macaw, Jabiru stork, jaguar, leopard, and the giant armadillo protected by the Endangered Species Act, CITES, and/or the Migratory Bird Treaty Act.[7] While Heredia had what appeared to be valid CITES permits to export certain tribal pieces with parts from Appendix II species, it was for educational purposes only and not for commercial sale. Also, import of the Appendix I species was not allowed, rendering a substantial portion of the collection illegal.

Both Small and Heredia received generous deals. Small pleaded guilty to a single misdemeanor violation of the Migratory Bird Treaty Act. Unlike Hrabobvsky's buyers, who'd paid minimal $2,000 to $5,000 fines, the Smithsonian secretary paid no fine and in January 2004 received two years' probation and one hundred hours of community service.[8] In addition, he forfeited his entire collection, worth at least the $400,000 he'd paid and emptying the $1.2 million private gallery that he'd had specially converted.

Heredia pleaded guilty to a Lacey Act felony. Despite her role as a dealer like Hrabovsky and selling collections of artifacts to Small and at least two other private collectors, she received credit under the federal sentencing guidelines for cooperating with government authorities. She also argued for a lighter sentence because of her hardship as a single parent and received just forty hours of community service, which the judge ordered that she spend preserving and protecting the Amazon.

While speaking generically, Hundley noted that for a successful prosecution "all things have to line up."[9] Good evidence is essential, as is a good prosecutor, a good court, and a good probation officer who writes the presentence report summarizing the case that the judge uses to set the penalty.

The mild sentences for Heredia and Small illustrate the lack of uniformity in sentencing for people who committed crimes like those of Hrabovsky and his clients. They also expose the low priority of wildlife crimes. Attorneys and law enforcement officials often regard wildlife trafficking as a minor infraction. In many countries, it is considered not a criminal offense but a civil violation that merits an administrative penalty and sometimes confiscation of the specimens. This minimal level of concern promotes the trade. Small's well-publicized collection, like the museum exhibits it came from, supplied a type of "official" sanction that persuaded others to follow suit and become collectors even though it was illegal. In interviews with FWS agents, several of Hrabovsky's buyers said the articles about Small's artifacts in *Smithsonian* magazine and again in *Architectural Digest* in December 2000 encouraged their own purchases and gave them confidence that what they were doing was legal. "Writing off" wildlife offenses with small slaps on the wrist lets the system, in essence, turn a blind eye to the crime. That tolerance allows everyone from dealers to prestigious institutions to private collectors to continue business as usual.

Fortunately, LeClair's case against Hrabovsky did more than just imprison a major dealer. It raised awareness about feather art within the law enforcement community and generated several new cases in the United States and Brazil.

FWS special agents, who number roughly two hundred, form a relatively small, cohesive community. They generally know about one another's cases and learn from other agents' experiences, but the Hrabovsky case directly involved agents across the country. There were defendants in almost every FWS region, so dozens of agents around the country had interviewed buyers. As a result, FWS law enforcement officers became sensitive to the problem of feathered artifact trafficking—and that led to more prosecutions.

In addition to the cases against Small and Heredia, in December 2004, FWS agents in Alaska investigated two people, Ray Reichmuth and Cynthia Brown, who operated a mall kiosk in Fairbanks that sold feathered and other artifacts illegally imported from Brazil. A search of the kiosk and residence resulted in confiscation of hundreds of items the lab identified as made from CITES and non-CITES species. The two, nicknamed "The Brazil Nuts," pleaded guilty and were given a $10,000 fine and sentenced to a lengthy probation term under the Endangered Species Act for unlawfully importing and selling tribal objects containing parts of endangered fish and wildlife from Brazil.

A similar case in Chicago in 2006 involved Glen Joffe and Claudia Ashleigh-Morgan, owners of Primitive Art Works, who stocked their upscale art gallery with illegally obtained ivory carvings, elaborate feathered Indian artifacts from the Amazon, and other items made from tiger, jaguar, hippopotamus, elephant, and sea turtle. Special Agent Matthew Bryant began investigating after a March 9, 2003, article in the Home and Garden section of the *Chicago Tribune* featured the pair and their collection. On April 21, 2003, when the couple returned from a buying trip to China, Customs agents at Chicago's O'Hare International Airport searched their baggage and found ivory carvings that Joffe said were made of bone and a sea turtle shell comb that Ashleigh-Morgan claimed was made of plastic. A search of their home two days later yielded $1 million worth of items containing threatened and endangered species and resulted in what prosecutors called "one of the largest seizures ever in the U.S. of such artifacts."[10] Of that, 72 items worth $175,000 were identified by the lab as containing protected migratory bird parts.[11] Both pleaded guilty to felony violations for smuggling protected animal products. Joffe received five years' probation and 1,500 hours of community service, and Ashleigh-Morgan received three years of probation, 600 hours of community service, and was fined $12,000.

Because of LeClair's connections with Brazilian authorities, Bryant and Brazilian federal police identified the couple's supplier, a French woman who smuggled artifacts from Brazil and to date has not been caught.[12]

The case against Hrabovsky laid the foundations for a consciousness among the general public, too. FWS and the Brazilian government donated most of the artifacts from the case to the Florida Museum of Natural History (at the University of Florida), under the condition that they not be bartered or sold by the museum, and that the museum publicly recognize that the items were illegally exported from Brazil for sale to collectors in the United States and Europe. Museum director of development Robert Hutchinson noted the donation would significantly expand its collection, especially because "there's no way we'd be able to get these things on our own" due to the ethical and legal issues preventing anthropologists from removing artifacts from the Amazon.[13] For its part, the museum planned to use the collection to educate the public about wildlife trafficking.

In addition, in November 2004 some of the artifacts and feathers from the Hrabovsky case that had been unambiguously identified were permanently transferred to the wildlife forensics lab for use as standards. These included some of the items destined for Sadofsky, the Rikbatsa Indian crown bought by LeClair, as well as six feathers belonging to his purchased Kamayura bow mask. It also included items seized from packages destined for Hrabovsky (a headdress, band, and cap with feathers) and others confiscated from Hrabovsky's properties such as a bone art item with six feather clusters including harpy eagle and scarlet macaw taken from the van outside one of the apartments, strands of Maguari stork and great egret feathers taken off a headdress confiscated from the storage facility, and strings of other feathers from harpy eagle, macaw, and other birds. This transfer of evidence provided the lab with many of the standards it had been lacking, and would facilitate identifications in future cases.

Perhaps the most significant impact of Hrabovsky's case, however, occurred in Brazil, where it disrupted a significant artifact-smuggling scheme. Brazilian authorities had encountered Hrabovsky in January 1999, but they had no clue about his operation until LeClair contacted them in November 2000 seeking clarification of that country's laws.

Jorge Pontes of Brazil's Federal Police—the country's national law enforcement arm that is akin to the U.S. Federal Bureau of Investigation (FBI), Drug Enforcement Agency (DEA), Immigration and Naturalization Service (INS), and Secret Service all rolled into one—became LeClair's key contact. Pontes was the Brazilian environmental federal police commissioner, the top environmental enforcement official in the country, and an unusual officer. He studied biology at college but quit that field to study law instead. At the age of twenty-six, he became a field investigator for the Brazilian Federal Police and at thirty-five became a chief (called *delegado*). He primarily focused on drug interdiction, white-collar crime, and protection details, and in the mid-1980s was sent to the Amazon. The Amazon touched him in a spiritual way, one that would inspire him to focus on protecting the rain forest's bountiful resources. The new awareness hit home when, during a routine drug search of a boat, he and his fellow agents found sixty giant freshwater turtles, each about the size of a sea turtle (over two feet long and weighing about fifty-five pounds). When one of the men in the boat dismissed the animals, saying "We have nothing—just turtles," Pontes couldn't help but think, "It wasn't 'nothing.'"

That event inspired Pontes to work toward the creation of a division in the federal police to fight against environmental crime. Beginning in 1996, he researched how other countries had done this and pressed for an agency like FWS. In 2001, the Brazilian Federal Police established its environmental crimes division (the Divisão de Repressão aos Crimes Ambientais, or DMAPH) with Pontes as its head. This case would be its first major investigation.

Hrabovsky's scheme was particularly distressing to Pontes. The magnitude of the dealings revealed itself over time as Pontes and LeClair exchanged information and investigated their respective pieces of the puzzle.

The collaboration had started with questions about permits for Hrabovsky's artifacts. While he knew Hrabovsky's imports into the United States were illegal, LeClair had also wanted to know the requirements from the Brazilian side for exporting featherwork. Official-looking tags had been attached to several of the artifacts, including two in the initial shipment confiscated at Dulles airport destined for Sadofsky and several uncovered by the mail covers. One of LeClair's questions was whether these tags were, in fact, permits and/or an official sanction of their sale.

Brazilian authorities said in a January 17, 2001, fax that the tags were "not valid as documents to cover the exportations"[14] and a June 12, 2002, communication explained further that the tags, labeled "Artindia" and "FUNAI," indicated the items were from the series of shops called Artindia supported by the National Indigenous Foundation (Fundação National do Índio), or FUNAI, a government agency within the Ministry of Justice that protects the interests of Brazil's Indians. They were simply sales tags that had descriptions of the item and sometimes a price.

While the tags imparted little except information about the seller, they were nonetheless significant. They proved these artifacts were supposed to be sold by FUNAI, not by another party or for export. As such, they provided the first inkling of a conspiracy to exploit Brazil's Amazonian Indians.

The ensuing investigation bolstered that suggestion. In early February 2003, LeClair met with Pontes in Roswell, New Mexico, while the Brazilian was attending a training session in the United States. The purpose of LeClair's meeting with Pontes was threefold: to establish a personal rapport; to clarify the Brazilian laws; and to better understand the meaning of the seized documents, some of which were written in Portuguese. Over the course of two days, in between Pontes's training, the Brazilian law enforcement officer explained the intricacies of the Brazilian laws and informally translated the files on suppliers and other documents. This initial meeting led to a deeper understanding of how Hrabovsky's operation worked and how the artifacts made their way to him from Brazil. It also provided Pontes with key documentation that would help his investigation, and gave him proof, from the FWS wildlife forensics lab, that the artifacts were illegal because they contained protected species.

The meeting confirmed that there was no legal way for someone to export CITES-regulated or endangered wildlife out of Brazil without proper CITES documents. Pontes's informal translation of Hrabovsky's correspondence further corroborated what Pontes considered a "conspiracy" to smuggle CITES-listed and endangered wildlife parts from Brazil. The records also indicated that FUNAI officials may have been involved, and generated an important line of investigation for Brazilian authorities.

After his return to Brazil in February 2003, Pontes launched a covert investigation into the suppliers called Operação (Operation) Pindo-rama.[15] He originally named it Operation LeClair to honor the FWS agent but the name had sounded too French so he changed it. Through the investigation, the Brazilian Federal Police learned the specifics of how Hrabovsky's scheme worked. Initially, Hrabovsky traded directly with Indian communities, exchanging $10 bags of used clothing for art that he'd spruce up with pristine feathers from captive-bred birds and sell for hundreds of dollars. Later, he dealt mostly with people running the FUNAI stores. It was easier for Hrabovsky that way. Brazilian law allowed the shipment of artifacts between its states, and FUNAI routinely bought and shipped between their stores, though not outside of the country. Like his clients, Hrabovsky reduced his own risk by distancing himself from the smuggling and letting the FUNAI officials do the buying for him. The government officials would buy the artifacts from the remote Amazonian tribes, transfer the material between stores, and then smuggle them via mail to America, where Hrabovsky and other dealers like Heredia turned a handsome profit.

Over the years, however, the scheme developed into something more exploitative. The Brazilian investigation found it had started in 1984.[16] Hrabovsky sent the FUNAI officials and other private merchants "grocery lists" of animal parts. The orders specified dozens of rare wildlife parts, including jaguar teeth and feathers from rare or endangered birds as well as parts from more common species such as monkeys and capybara (the largest rodent in the world that is related to guinea pigs and can grow to over four feet long). Indians were then paid a minimal amount to fill the orders, and undertook special hunts specifically for that purpose.

In Brazil, Indian art crafts that are sold are supposed to be constructed using "leftover" parts from animals that indigenous groups hunted for other reasons, such as food, clothing, and ceremonies. In this case, however, the animals were killed only to supply the artifact market. Even worse, the Indians didn't make the feathered pieces that Hrabovsky sold as "authentic." Brazilian investigators found that once his orders for wholesale parts were filled, either Hrabovsky or the merchants would fabricate the "Indian" artifact.

In May 2004, Pontes and the Brazilian police closed their covert investigation. During the takedown, Brazilian Federal Police executed search warrants in seven states (Rondônia, Amapá, Pará, Mato

Grosso, Goiás, the Federal District, and São Paulo) and over a dozen cities across Brazil, including Brasilia, Manaus, Belém, Altamira, Porto Velho, Cuibá, Maraba, and Sâo Félix do Araguaia, among others. In each state, they targeted several people. They raided Artindia shops in Belém, Cuiabá, Manaus, Recife, São Paulo, and Rio de Janeiro as well as private shops such as Amoa Konoya Arte Indígena with stores in São Paulo and São Félix do Araguaia.

The result included the arrest of eleven people, including seven FUNAI officials who ran stores in at least three states (Pará, Rondônia, and Mato Grosso), and several owners of private shops.

On April 10, 2008, Brazil made its first conviction stemming from the Brazilian investigation, of Lilaz de Souza Loureiro from Belém in the state of Pará for illegally exporting rare wild animal parts under the guise of Native workmanship. The evidence seized by LeClair as well as the species identifications made by the lab were instrumental in making the case against him. Because de Souza Loureiro had been prosecuted previously for smuggling and selling illegal goods, he faces a possible three to fifteen years' imprisonment.

Despite the arrests and this conviction, illegal trade in Indian artifacts continues. In July 2008, one of the people arrested in conjunction with Operation Pindorama, eighty-year-old Noel Rachid from São Felix do

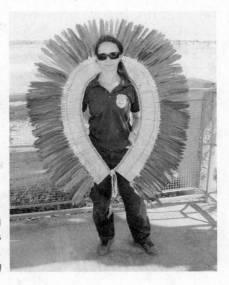

Brazilian Federal Police agent holding a headdress made of macaw feathers seized in Operation Pindorama.
(Courtesy of Brazilian Federal Police)

Araguaia, was again arrested for illegally selling Indian artifacts made from animal parts and faced a penalty of six months to a year in prison.

Operation Pindorama led to the seizure of over four thousand artifacts, each evaluated by the Brazilian Federal Police forensics laboratory and made of numerous parts from Brazil's threatened and endangered wild fauna. One of the most deplorable examples, for Pontes, was a jaguar tooth necklace made with forty-four canines from at least eleven separate animals.

In Brazil, the case generated a great deal of media attention, including by TV Centroamérica, Jornal Livre, Araguaia News, Ecol News, Globo.com, JB Online, *Cinform,* Ambiente Brasil, and Fauna Brasil, among others. The scheme was seen as a travesty in terms of government corruption and the exploitation of animals and Indians.

In 2004, the law changed as a result of this investigation. After Pontes testified before the Brazilian Congress, the president of FUNAI, Mercio Pereira Gomes, forbade the sale of all artifacts with animal parts. No one could openly sell these artifacts. Following this order,

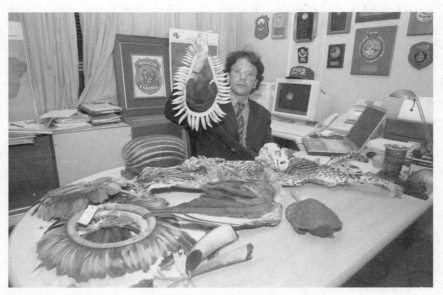

Brazilian Federal Police commissioner Jorge Pontes holding a necklace made of jaguar teeth seized in Operation Pindorama. *(Courtesy of Brazilian Federal Police)*

federal police all over Brazil went through shops to look for violations. While store owners continue to pressure the government to change this restriction, for now it remains in place. As Pontes later said, the animals are at least "free of one more kind of pressure."[17]

LeClair and Pontes's collaboration was unusual in that it was the first time an FWS case agent worked with foreign government officials of that ranking. Previously, bilateral cooperation occurred at higher levels, and the FWS agent had to go through his or her supervisor, who sought approval from the State Department, before contact occurred. U.S. and foreign law enforcement agents had rarely developed the personal connections necessary to exchange information freely and in a timely manner. But the open avenue for communication facilitated the investigations in both countries, enhancing each man's ability to pursue his case. Pontes gained access to FWS evidence and expertise and in return he held his case until LeClair served the search warrants on Hrabovsky. The cooperation and exchange of information was vital to both parties. LeClair solidified his case against Hrabovsky, and Brazilian authorities furthered their parallel investigation. Ultimately, it led to the disruption of a significant artifact smuggling scheme.

In late January 2005, Brazil sent a three-person delegation consisting of Pontes, Congressman Antonio Carlos Mendez Thame, a leading politician against biopiracy, and a FUNAI official who was in charge of one of the Artindia shops that the Brazilian police had searched, to meet with FWS law enforcement officers, including LeClair, at the agent's FWS office in Sandusky, Ohio. The intention was to allow the Brazilian delegation to discuss smuggling issues and to photograph and document all of the Brazilian tribal artifacts evidence that had been seized or abandoned, but it also served another key purpose: to educate the congressman and FUNAI official about the extent of the commercialization of Brazilian natural resources.

To illustrate this point, LeClair and his colleagues had filled the FWS conference room with dozens of tables and laid out the more than one thousand artifacts related to the Hrabovsky investigation that had been seized or abandoned during the case.

The display filled a fifty-foot-long room, and each table was crammed with artifact after artifact, each beautiful and unique, and the message hit home. The breadth of the exploitation stunned the dignitaries. The display was the output of only one dealer, and it encompassed only his known dealings. If others were doing the same, the potential smuggling of Brazilian Amazonian Indian patrimony was staggering.

This impression was reinforced a few days later (January 26–28, 2005) when Special Agent LeClair and the Brazilian delegation traveled from Ohio to Florida to talk with a number of people involved in the Hrabovsky and Heredia cases, who had also purchased artifacts from the same FUNAI officials. With Assistant U.S. Attorney McMahon (who'd prosecuted Hrabovsky) assisting, the delegation interviewed Heredia, who admitted the full extent of her dealings. Following up on that conversation, Brazilian agents subsequently raided her parents' home in Brazil, where she'd stored her illicit handicrafts, and seized two thousand more items.

Combining Hrabovsky's activities with Heredia's and the seven FUNAI officials, the size of this "known" artifact smuggling ring was likely around $12 million. Authorities estimate that less than half of one percent of Brazil's illegal wildlife trafficking is successfully intercepted

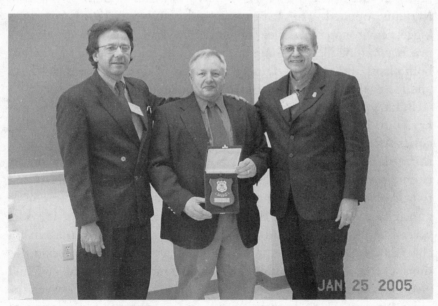

Brazilian Federal Police commissioner Jorge Pontes, USFWS special agent Daniel LeClair, and Brazilian congressman Antonio Carlos Mendez Thame meet in Ohio. *(Courtesy of Daniel LeClair)*

by the police,[18] and it is likely that other gangs operate similar schemes. If even only eight or nine others existed, the size of the Indian artifact market would be on the order of $100 million.

To show their colleagues the extent and potential impact of illegal wildlife smuggling, the Brazilian delegation brought the evidence home. They videotaped every item LeClair had laid out and even took representative samples, about fifteen of the nicer artifacts, back to Brazil to show the Brazilian Congress and government departments exactly what was being smuggled out of the country. The FWS wildlife forensics lab's findings on the artifacts made it impossible to ignore the number and range of species involved.

The exposure intensified environmental enforcement and raised awareness about the theft of Brazil's wild resources, which, in turn, led to increased political and budgetary support of the environmental crime unit and training for its officers. As a result of this and other cases (like the breaking of a ring of timber traffickers and shutting down their illegal sawmills in 2004),[19] the environmental crime unit that Pontes headed was strengthened. In November 2004, a new environmental police academy deep in Brazil's rain forest, four hours upriver from Manaus, opened. The 135-square-mile facility is Latin America's biggest environmental police training camp. At it, federal police officers practice raiding illegal mining or logging sites and stopping the theft of both plants and animals, training designed to enforce the country's laws and lower the illegal export of Brazil's patrimony.

Brazil's police agents also received training from FWS. From February 14 to 25, 2005, FWS, with funding from the U.S. embassy's Narcotics Affairs Section, held a training workshop in Brasilia, Brazil, for thirty-three federal agents from police headquarters in each of the twenty-seven states, as well as two representatives from FUNAI and two from IBAMA, on combating environmental crimes. The course aimed to raise awareness that wildlife trafficking in Brazil is widespread and extends beyond Brazil's borders; to train special agents in charge (*delegados*) on methods to disrupt wildlife criminal organizations; to share the information, intelligence, and experience of FWS and also that of the participants; and to facilitate cooperation between the federal police, FUNAI, and IBAMA and encourage coordination of their efforts to combat wildlife trafficking. The course was such a success that FWS repeated it in 2006.

With its forensics lab providing crucial support for prosecutions, today, according to Pontes, who now heads Interpol in Brazil, the environmental crime unit is the most important division in Brazil's Federal Police.[20]

At a time when deforestation from agricultural expansion, road construction, and other development projects already threaten the rain forest, animal trafficking adds yet another stress to an already stressed system.

According to Dener Giovanini, coordinator of the Brazilian Network to Combat the Wild Animal Trafficking (RENCTAS), a Brazilian nongovernmental wildlife trade monitoring organization, animal trafficking has unexpected consequences. "What we are seeing is a still-unknown level of damage to the most important ecosystem in the world. You cannot drain the Amazon of its life and expect it to keep functioning normally," he said.[21]

The huge volume of illegal trade represents thousands of Amazonian animals. With a single artifact containing feathers from as many as five bird species, every thousand artifacts could represent as many as five thousand different birds that were killed.[22] Each of those birds plays a critical role in the ecosystem and their removal affects the plants and animals that depend on them. However, we don't yet know exactly how the reduction or removal of certain kinds of birds, which represent over 80 percent of Brazil's illegal wildlife trafficking, will impact the Amazon rain forest. The likelihood, however, is that when they are no longer around to serve as seed dispersers, seed predators, and pest controllers, the ecosystem will be affected at every level.

Despite Brazil's mandate for a crackdown on wildlife trafficking, some of the most rigorous environmental laws of all developing countries and better training for enforcement, Brazilian agents face bigger obstacles. Deforestation is such an overwhelming problem for Amazonian wildlife that every other issue takes a backseat.

Deforestation from agriculture, ranching, and logging has already shrunk the rain forest by as much as 20 percent, and it may worsen. Plans to pave the 600 miles of the 1,100-mile dirt road that is the main north-south artery through the Amazon (called BR-163) without adequate safeguards and policing would, according to Brazilian environment minister Marina Silva in 2004, destroy a 62-mile-wide swath along its entire length.[23] That's a lot of land—over 37,000 square miles. Similarly, the government's proposal to build seven dams on major Amazon River tributaries would both alter the surrounding ecology and expand road construction, both of which would further the destruction of the forest.

While some people, such as Blairo Maggi, Brazil's leading soybean producer and the governor of Mato Grosso State, which alone accounts for 40 percent of the Amazon's deforestation, assert that "deforestation is an overblown issue, a 'phobia' that plagues people who can't grasp the enormity of the Amazon,"[24] environmentalists, scientists, and others say the problem could reach a tipping point where the situation could fly out of control, as happened in Brazil's Atlantic rain forest.

The Atlantic rain forest was once a third the size of the Amazon. But 97 percent of it was wiped out when it became, in the words of Environment Minister Silva in 2004, "just another resource deposit for our economic demands."[25] A similar threat exists in the Amazon, where people like slash-and-burn farmers, ranchers, rubber tappers, loggers, and soybean producers exploit it for their livelihood and financial gain.

With huge profits to be made from wildlife trafficking, its low priority and limited resources allocation vis-à-vis deforestation, environmental law enforcement in Brazil faces an uphill battle in slowing these illegal activities across a continent-sized area. As Jorge Pontes has put it, fighting environmental crimes in the Amazon "is like changing a tire on a moving car."[26]

The lab is a vital tool to fight that crime. But as long as it is more profitable to destroy the Amazon—by embezzling the cultural heritage of its people, stealing its wildlife, or cutting it down for short-term grazing and farming—than to leave it standing, then that's what will happen.

CHAPTER TEN

Conclusion

When television satirist Stephen Colbert asked on *The Colbert Report,* "Do we need *all* the animals? A lot of them are similar. Do we need tigers *and* lions? Crocodiles *and* alligators?"[1] he playfully highlighted the importance of individual species. But the phrasing of his question also highlighted that the existence of many animals is dependent on whether humans deem them necessary. They must have value to us. Too often, their value consists only of the products they provide. In our consumer culture, we value ivory knickknacks, bear bile, and feather art more than we do the animals that provide them.

We also don't think about the effect of our demand for these products. But demand is a powerful force. Any wildlife special agent will tell you that if nobody wanted these illicit and rare items, they'd be out of work. Unfortunately, their job prospects are good.

As with most crimes, the scale of illegal wildlife trafficking is dependent on the risk-reward trade-off. Strong consumer demand for illicit wildlife products equals large profits for traffickers, while the risks they face are often modest at best.

The extremely lucrative markets for illicit wildlife products are irresistible to many—more so than following the law. Compared to the huge prospective income, punishments for wildlife trafficking, such as fines or the confiscation of the illegal items, tend to be little more than an annoying "tax" that barely dents the smuggler's overall business. In the United States, a 1994 study on the FWS wildlife inspection program by the General Accounting Office (GAO) noted that only a quarter of violators of the Endangered Species Act received any penalty, with a far lower percentage sentenced to probation or prison. Even repeat offenders rarely received substantial fines or jail time.[2]

Minimal punishments for wildlife trafficking are also common in other countries. In Japan, a prime destination for illicit elephant ivory, a recent smuggling case involving 1 billion yen ($9.4 million) worth of raw and worked ivory resulted in an 800,000-yen ($7,500) fine, less than one-tenth of one percent of the value of the consignment.[3] In Thailand, a Bangkok luxury store owner selling $20,000 of illegal shahtoosh shawls received two years' probation and a $300 fine,[4] while in Indonesia, a major trafficker of rhino horn and tiger bone and skins who'd operated with impunity for almost two decades received only an eighteen-month jail sentence—and his partners and clients escaped any sort of reprimand.[5] These nominal penalties show that prosecutors, judges, police, and policy makers are not terribly concerned about crimes against wildlife.

The low priority given to wildlife crimes leaves the responsible enforcement agencies underfunded[6] and understaffed. According to the CITES Secretariat, the failure of many countries to consider wildlife offenses a "serious, high-value, 'mainstream' crime"[7] prevents enforcement agencies from accessing the human, technological, and forensic science assistance needed for investigations and results in governments enacting policies and laws "without allocating the necessary financial resources to implement them."[8]

The lack of funding affects staffing at every level of wildlife enforcement. At the international level, only two law enforcement officers are employed full-time—one at the CITES Secretariat and one at Interpol—even though much illicit wildlife trade occurs across national borders.

At the national level, resources are equally scarce. In the United States, which is one of the world's largest markets for illegal wildlife products and a major source of supply, roughly 200 federal wildlife special agents and 3,300 state wildlife game wardens police a country of 300 million people. Compare that number to over 12,000 Federal Bureau of Investigation special agents (with 200 agents and support staff stationed overseas),[9] more than 5,000 Drug Enforcement Administration special agents,[10] and roughly 675,000 sworn state and local police officers.[11]

FWS wildlife inspectors, a force of just under 115 officers stationed at seventeen designated ports[12] with limited coverage at twenty other locations, are the first line of defense against wildlife crimes. Compare that to the U.S. Customs and Border Patrol, which has 33,000 border patrol agents, officers, and agriculture specialists to detect illegal immigrants and contraband at points of entry into the country.[13]

Wildlife inspectors are overwhelmed because they must detect illegal wildlife and products smuggled in cargo and personal baggage and also clear the more than 187,600 legitimate wildlife shipments worth $2.8 billion that enter and leave the country each year.[14] Of the 20,000 containers that come into the major ports like Los Angeles and New York each day, generally fewer than 20 are inspected.[15] Supervisory Wildlife Inspector Robert Onda, a wildlife inspection veteran since 1975, described the overload: "We must identify thousands of species in all forms and know the requirements for each. . . . We can't keep up with the volume even with weekend and overtime work."[16] Jorge Picon, a senior FWS enforcement agent in Miami, agreed and noted that his five inspectors in Miami were "enough to examine 3% of wildlife shipments for contraband."[17]

A similar refrain can be heard among wildlife law enforcement agencies around the world: staffing levels are tiny compared to the need. In England, Scotland Yard's wildlife crime unit consists of only one four-person team.[18] In Belém, Brazil, a major hub for illegal wildlife trade from the Amazon, sixty IBAMA agents monitor trafficking in wild plants and animals for the entire state of Pará—a huge area that makes up one-sixth of the country. They also inspect incoming containers and luggage at the city's massive port and international airport.[19] "Of course there are more smugglers out there than we can catch, and that is frustrating," Lucimar Paixao, manager of IBAMA's Belém fauna division, said. "But we're doing the best we can with what we have."[20]

The U.S. Fish and Wildlife Service Forensics Laboratory helps these overstressed agencies do more with what they have. It has changed the face of wildlife law enforcement by allowing prosecutors to prove beyond a reasonable doubt when a smuggled animal product is, in fact, illegal. Without that corroboration, agents can't always prove a crime occurred. Instead of needing eyewitnesses or agents to track the contraband from its origin through production to a final point of sale, the lab teases the story out of the evidence. And that is "worth another one hundred agents in the field."[21]

The lab also enhances agents' effectiveness by letting them focus their efforts higher up the supply chain—that is, on the commercial market for parts and products of rare animals. For example, rather than concentrating on catching sturgeon poachers, who operate in remote locales and are easily replaced by others, agents pursue illegal caviar traders who are the real motivation behind the illegal killing. Ultimately, this tactic can have a greater impact.

Wildlife forensics helps law enforcement agencies work smarter and target their limited resources. The lab's insights into criminals' methods, such as mislabeling caviar or using poisoned calves as bait for wolves, make it easier for agents to prevent future crimes. This exposure can revolutionize thinking about how illicit trafficking networks operate and improve law enforcement's approach. Recent DNA analysis of massive illegal elephant ivory shipments (6.5 tons seized in Singapore in 2002 and 3.9 tons confiscated in Hong Kong in 2006), conducted by a team headed by Dr. Samuel Wasser, director of the Center for Conservation Biology at the University of Washington (with help from the lab), showed that the ivory came from closely related elephants from specific localities (eastern Zambia for the Singapore seizure and a small section of eastern Gabon and neighboring Congo for the Hong Kong one).[22] These results indicated that, rather than collecting ivory from disparate sources as was previously thought, organized gangs filled "purchase orders" by targeting whole herds at particular sites. That information will help antipoaching units center their patrols on precise geographic areas and allow agents to monitor little-known but well-worn smuggling routes.

The lab plays a vital role not just for FWS agents but also for enforcement worldwide. Cases ranging from the Canadian bear gallbladders to Amazonian feather art to caviar and shahtoosh shawls demonstrate how the lab's impact extends beyond U.S. borders. The lab's impact is felt not only each time it analyzes evidence but also each time its identification protocols are employed by wildlife forensic scientists around the world. Its effectiveness has also inspired other countries, including Mexico, India, and Kenya, to explore the establishment of wildlife crime sections within their national forensic laboratories.

The lab must constantly evolve to anticipate future trends in wildlife trafficking. As poachers and smugglers find new species to target or new products come on the black market, the wildlife forensics lab must develop strategies to cope with the forensic and legal challenges before they happen.

Just as the lab had to develop a protocol for testing bear bile, it will also have to obtain standards and discover defining traits each time a new species becomes so threatened by commercial trade that it is given legal protection. Sharks, sea horses, and tropical timber are but a few of the examples of the range of species and problems facing the lab in the near term. Because some shark species are rare and because there are so many different kinds of sharks (over four hundred species of sharks and rays), collecting shark fins to use as standards is problematic. Identification of sea horses is tricky because no one knows the total number of species and because scientists don't yet understand how habitat, locality, temperature, or age affect variations in color, size, and form. And expansion of the lab's work into tropical timber will present its own challenges.

While the lab's mandate has always included plants (and it has been involved in wild American ginseng cases), most of its work has concentrated on animals. That's because of the extensive legal protections for animals. Yet that may change. In May 2008, amendment of the Lacey Act made it illegal to import, export, transport, buy, or sell any plant or plant product that was illegally taken or traded. With the United States the world's largest importer of wood and wood products, and much of that illegally harvested, the lab may soon be called on to identify illicit timber.

In addition to discovering the unique traits of additional species, the lab will also need to untangle issues of timing and geographic origin in order to stay ahead of the legal curve. Legal protections are often contingent on the date when a species became protected. Therefore, knowing whether the animal in a piece of evidence died or was imported before or after the date when it became protected is crucial for determining if a crime was committed. Remember that this is why LeClair spent so much time verifying exactly when Hrabovsky imported his artifacts.

Determining exact dates from animal parts and processed pieces requires expensive equipment and expertise that the lab doesn't possess. It currently relies on the Lawrence Livermore National Laboratory in Livermore, California, to date products using carbon-14 ratios (which are tied to degradation over time). However, the testing is expensive, though not as expensive as buying the same equipment, making it critical for the lab to find other ways of establishing exact dates.

Because legal protections increasingly may become not just species-specific but species- *and* location-specific, the geographic origins of species are another growing area of inquiry for the lab. When trade regulations vary for different geographic populations of the same species, the lab can determine the legality of a product by isolating its origin. For example, the lab can use location to distinguish between captive-bred pet birds, which are legal, and wild-caught ones, which are not.

DNA analysis can provide clues to the geographic origin of evidence. Yet extraction of DNA is difficult, and more important, scientists must have something to compare the DNA to. Without the ability to weigh the evidence against a range of known standards, scientists cannot identify where the specimen came from.

Currently, the lab's Genetics Standards Collection contains over 40,000 samples from more than 800 mammal species, 600 bird species, 50 fish species, and 100 amphibian and reptile species. Much of its extensive reference collection comes from North American taxa, partly because it's easier to obtain samples locally. The lab's collection of DNA from bears, for example, started in the early 1990s and has continued with agents still sending tissue samples. This large data set now allows the lab to tell with ease whether a bear part (including a gallbladder when a bit of liver is attached) came from the Smoky Mountains or Yosemite.[23] They are able to do the same for deer, eagles, and wolves.

When the lab doesn't have a comprehensive DNA database, it can't make these types of identifications. For many kinds of animals, such as reptiles, which comprise over 8,700 species, the lab does not have a robust collection of reference samples, particularly for foreign specimens. Obtaining enough samples can be difficult, especially when populations are small, as in the case of rare and endangered species. It's also problematic when there are many related species, as in the case of sharks. Yet without an extensive DNA reference collection, the lab can't always resolve the legal issue. Therefore, the lab is exploring other methods to isolate the geographic origin of evidence, such as isotope analysis.

Keeping ahead of illegal traffickers also requires adequate numbers of wildlife forensic scientists. With almost every new case now involv-

ing digital evidence, the lab is increasing its number of computer forensic specialists. If illegal plant trafficking cases become significant, the lab
will also need to hire a botanist. Training the next generation of morphologists is probably the most critical staffing challenge facing the
wildlife forensics lab. Currently, no university trains forensic morphologists, so the lab has established a master-apprenticeship program
whereby an apprentice learns at the side of a master scientist for five
years.

Over time, however, wildlife forensics as a unique field will likely
grow, with the consequent expansion in jobs and training. Already, the
American Society of Crime Lab Directors' Laboratory Accreditation
Board has accredited the U.S. Fish and Wildlife Service Forensics Lab,
which validates its professionalism and gives the field additional standing among other forensic scientists, and the International Association
of Forensic Sciences has recognized wildlife forensics as a new field of
science.[24] For all of the high-tech equipment available to the lab, nothing can ever substitute for human expertise.

While the U.S. Fish and Wildlife Service Forensics Laboratory has
improved the effectiveness of wildlife law enforcement and raised the
risks to traffickers, more is needed. Significantly reducing illicit wildlife
trade also requires shifting the incentives that encourage the trafficking
in the first place.

When consumers and sellers value animals only for the products they
can provide, wildlife will continue to be exploited and possibly endangered. Once people value the sustainability of future populations, the
calculus changes so that animals are worth more alive than dead.

On the supply side, those living close to the targeted animals should
profit from wildlife conservation. Many win-win situations already
create economic incentives to conserve wildlife and its habitat while
allowing sustainable utilization. In southern Africa, for example, communities that live near national parks and hunting areas in Botswana,
Namibia, Zambia, and elsewhere make money off elephants, lions,
zebras, and other wildlife by selling limited hunting quotas and/or
through ecotourism. For them, it has become more profitable to preserve the animals than to kill them. Scarlet macaws and other bird
species have a similar potential to attract tourists and money. And
Native Alaskan communities could follow this model of generating rev-

enue from species' conservation by creating a "brand" for sustainably caught or produced products, as has been done for fair-trade timber and shade-grown coffee. Carved or scrimshawed ivory could be officially labeled as a product of sustainable subsistence hunting and be sold at a premium price. However, for a "subsistence hunting label" to work, consumers must be confident that limited catches do not hurt the overall population.

We must also reduce demand from those at the end of the supply chain. Consumers can help stem the tide through awareness of animal trafficking and consciousness of what they purchase. As in the campaign against fur or the outcry against diamonds during the height of apartheid, or blood diamonds more recently, when consumers' tastes change, they can reduce demand and shift a product toward substitutes.

Conservation must be made more attractive than poaching and illegal trafficking. The lab's ability to reveal the source of that illegal ivory pendant, shahtoosh shawl, or traditional medicine helps punish the trader directly and also makes buyers aware of what they're getting. That, in turn, can make the product less desirable to consumers, lowering its price and, as a consequence, the profitability of poaching and trafficking.

When individuals, communities, and politicians value wildlife conservation, law enforcement becomes that much easier. Each of the lab's victories is a significant step toward stopping crimes against wildlife— and ultimately conserving endangered species.

While the public can advocate for more enforcement, bears can't protest. And dead birds can't complain.

The victims of wildlife crimes are silent, but the wildlife forensics lab gives them a voice—one that grows stronger every day. Yet it's up to us to sustain their ability to speak.

ACKNOWLEDGMENTS

I'm privileged to have been aided by so many remarkable people during this writing adventure. I'm sincerely grateful to Steve Osofsky, a wildlife veterinarian whose friendship and intuition sparked and supported this incredible journey.

This book would not have been possible without the enthusiasm, cooperation, and patience of the many talented scientists at the U.S. Fish and Wildlife Service Forensics Laboratory. The welcome of lab director Ken Goddard was invaluable, as were his insights, humor, and words of praise along the way. Deputy director Ed Espinoza also provided countless hours of patient explanation as well as a window into the perspective of a forensic scientist, for which I am eternally grateful. Pepper Trail awed me with his passion and talent, and I greatly appreciate his passing on to me the wonder of how an animal's parts reflect their form and function. Many others currently or previously at the lab also provided indispensable assistance, including Verlin Cross, Mary Curtis, Darrell Hegdahl, Pam McClure, Darby Morrell, Mike Scanlan, Jo Ann Shafer, Cookie Sims, Dick Stroud, Doina Voin, and Bonnie Yates, among others. While not employed by the lab, another scientist, Lee Hagey, warmly offered a seemingly endless supply of good humor and plain speaking that I valued tremendously.

Numerous special agents and others currently or previously serving with the U.S. Fish and Wildlife Service's Office of Law Enforcement helped immeasurably with my efforts. The list is long and I cannot hope to thank these amazing people in a way that truly reflects their help and support. Sandy Cleva cheerfully supplied answers to my abundant questions, including contacts with the undercover and other agents who worked on these cases. Al Crane's initial words of discouragement clearly didn't work and I relied on his insights throughout. Winning him over was one of my greatest accomplishments, and I deeply value our enduring friendship. Mark Webb opened his heart and enthusiasm to help me understand the issues at stake. Dan LeClair, too, provided incalculable assistance and his dedication not only makes the world a better place but made this book a better one. My sincerest thanks go to Salvatore Amato, Matt Bryant, Marion Dean, Terry Grosz, Allen Hundley, George Morrison, Steve Oberholtzer, Benito Perez, Kim Speckman, Suzann Speckman, Bob Standish, Mike Wade, and other unnamed agents of the U.S. Fish and Wildlife Service, all of whom are still currently working to protect wildlife resources. Chris Servheen deserves special mention for sharing his incredible knowledge of issues surrounding trade in bear parts and bear conservation and, in so doing, inspiring me and hopefully also the readers of this book.

In northwestern Alaska, many warmly shared their hospitality, coffee, and insights into subsistence hunting and the Native culture. I would especially like to thank the Eskimo Walrus Commission, the Qayassiq Walrus Commission, Tom and Shirley Antoghame, Leonard Apangalook, Edmond Apassingok, Helen Chythlook, Timothy Dyasuk, Linda Jeschke, Victor Karmun, Vera Metcalf, Beulah Oittilliah, Aaron Oseuk, Erna and Leo Rasmussen, Martin Robards, Frank and Judith Stein, and others who would prefer not to be mentioned.

In British Columbia, Canada, Rod Olsen spent long hours explaining the intricacies of bear gall trafficking in the province and the specifics of the undercover case that he spearheaded. I'm also grateful for the detailed remembrances, perspectives, and friendly encouragement of Mike Girard, Dan LeGrandeur, Ralph Krenz, and James MacAulay.

In Brazil, Jorge Pontes's devotion to the animals and environment reinforced my belief in the potential of this book to affect the perspective of its readers. I'm eternally appreciative of his warm reception, comprehensive description of the Brazilian side of the Amazonian Indian feather art investigation, and willingness to answer all of my questions until I'd exhausted them, particularly given his pressing duties as the current head of Interpol in Brazil.

Many others also invested countless hours sharing their stories and helping me understand their complexities, including Tommy Dades, Jill Robinson, and Skip Wissinger. I greatly appreciate their time and openness. I also wish to thank Bill Clark, Adam Mekler, Cristina G. Mittermeier, Patrick Omondi, Ron Orenstein, Wayne Pacelle, Adam Roberts, Kent Redford, John Sellar, Teresa Telecky, Sam Wasser, and Louisa Willcox for their assistance in broadening the picture.

My editor at Scribner, Samantha Martin, provided sensitivity, enthusiasm, and guidance that made this book stronger and the process exciting and fun. I'd also like to express my sincere thanks to Susan Moldow, Nan Graham, Tyler LeBleu, Heidi Richter, and the rest of the Scribner team. My agent, Jeff Kleinman of Folio Literary Management, gave me exceptional guidance and support that made this book possible, and I am eternally grateful for his assistance. I also express my heartfelt appreciation to Richard Leakey and Jane Goodall for their belief in and support of this effort.

Finally, thanks to friends and family, especially Meryl Abrams, Karen Alvarenga, Patty Bliss, Janice Foley, and Kimberly Jessup, who have been great sources of encouragement. Cheryl Dorschner provided heartening words of wisdom in the bleakest times, Jack Heffron gave me advice and encouragement, and Kevin Clayton at Village Wine & Coffee gave me a friendly "home" away from home. I'm particularly grateful for the kindness of Ann and Joe Neme, who supplied their caring grandparenting services when I most needed it so that I could travel to research this book. My mother, Isabel Abrams, brainstormed and edited many rough drafts and consistently reassured me that I could do it while my father and hero, Allen Abrams, showed me through example that one has to be true to one's heart, despite the apparent lack of monetary gain. My husband and soul mate, Chris, supported me in every way—emotionally, professionally, and financially—while our wonderful and full-of-wonder son, Jackson, was my greatest cheerleader. Jackson's unique perspective helped keep me on track and deepened my dedication to this project. I am blessed by this bounty of care and love.

While I have tried to be as accurate as possible and verify material with the sources, all errors are strictly my own.

NOTES

Introduction

1. Ben Davies, *Black Market: Inside the Endangered Species Trade in Asia* (San Rafael, Calif.: Earth Aware Editions, 2005), p. 27.
2. International Fund for Animal Welfare, *Killing with Keystrokes: An Investigation of the Illegal Wildlife Trade on the World Wide Web* (Yarmouth Port, Mass., 2008), p. 9.
3. "Environmental Crimes: Profiting at the Earth's Expense," *Environmental Health Perspectives* 112, No. 2 (February 2004). See www.ehponline.org/mem bers/2004/112–2/focus.html.
4. Ibid.
5. Statement of William Clark before the U.S. House of Representatives, Committee on Natural Resources, March 5, 2008, p. 3.
6. Sharon Begley, "Extinction Trade: Endangered Animals Are the New Blood Diamonds as Militias and Warlords Use Poaching to Fund Death," *Newsweek,* March 10, 2008.
7. Statement of John A. Hart, scientific director, Tshuapa-Lomami-Lualaba Project, Democratic Republic of Congo, before the Committee on Natural Resources, U.S. House of Representatives, Hearing on "Poaching American Security: Impacts of Illegal Wildlife Trade," March 5, 2008.
8. Adrian Levy and Cathy Scott-Clark, "Poaching for Bin Laden," *The Guardian,* May 5, 2007. See www.guardian.co.uk/world/2007/may/05/terrorism.animal welfare.
9. Statement of Representative Nick J. Rahall II, Chairman, House Committee on Natural Resources, Hearing on "Poaching American Security: Impacts of Illegal Wildlife Trade," March 5, 2008.
10. Davies, *Black Market,* p. 55.
11. Ibid., p. 37.
12. Liana Sun Wyler and Pervaze Sheikh, *International Trade in Wildlife: Threats and U.S. Policy,* Congressional Research Service Report for Congress, Washington, D.C., March 3, 2008, p. 7.
13. Begley, "Extinction Trade."
14. Testimony of Claudia A. McMurray, assistant secretary, Bureau of Oceans, Environment and Science, U.S. Department of State, before the Committee on Natural Resources, U.S. House of Representatives, Hearing on "Poaching American Security: Impacts of Illegal Wildlife Trade," March 5, 2008.
15. Ibid., www.state.gov/g/oes/rls/rm/101794.htm.
16. Davies, *Black Market,* p. 21.
17. "The Feather Trade and the American Conservation Movement," a virtual exhi-

bition from the Smithsonian Institution's National Museum of American History, https://americanhistory.si.edu/feather/ftintxt.htm.

18. Davies, *Black Market,* p. 60.

19. Peter H. Sand, "Whither CITES? The Evolution of a Treaty Regime in the Borderland of Trade and Environment," *European Journal of International Law* 8, no. 1 (1997), pp. 3–4.

20. "Trade: Reptile Trade: Crocodiles and Alligators," *Endangered Species Handbook,* Segment 323, www.endangeredspecieshandbook.org/trade_reptile_ croco diles.php.

21. Information compiled using data from FWS Division of Law Enforcement Annual Reports. Data is through FY2007.

22. Jon R. Luoma, "The Wild World's Scotland Yard," *Audubon,* November/December 2000, p. 76.

23. Barbara Sleeper, "Scotland Yard for Wildlife," *Animals,* September/October 1993, p. 15.

24. Author interview with Terry Grosz, August 9, 2004.

25. Richard Willing, "Prosecutors' Latest Tool: Animal DNA," *USA Today,* November 7, 2002, p. 24A.

Chapter One: Native Alaskan Subsistence Hunting

1. David F. Pelly, *Sacred Hunt* (Vancouver, B.C.: Greystone Books, 2001), p. 106.

2. Martin Robards and Julie Lurman Joly, "Interpretation of 'Wasteful Manner' Within the Marine Mammal Protection Act and Its Role in Management of the Pacific Walrus," *Ocean and Coastal Law Journal* 13, no. 2 (2008), p. 206.

3. People had long sought elephant ivory for everything from piano keys to jewelry. Yet legal and illegal ivory trade nearly decimated the African elephant population. In just ten years, hunting for ivory nearly halved the African elephant population (and killed perhaps as many as 80 percent of East African elephants), with numbers plummeting from 1.3 million animals in 1979 to 750,000 in 1989, and shrinking further to between 300,000 and 600,000 in 1995. In response, the Convention on International Trade in Endangered Species (CITES) banned trade in elephant ivory in 1989. While illegal poaching continued, customers also turned to substitutes, like bone, plastic, and animal teeth, as replacements.

4. See www.canadianivory.com/#walrus.

5. EWC represents nineteen walrus-hunting communities, including: Barrow, Brevig Mission, Clarks Point, Gambell, Kivalina, Kings Island, Kotzebue, Kwigillingok, Little Diomede, Mekoryuk, Nome, Point Hope, Point Lay, Savoonga, Shishmaref, Stebbins, Unalakleet, Wainwright, and Wales.

6. While neither Asigrook nor Crane could remember their exact words, they both agree that Asigrook's words, recorded by NBC's *Dateline* for their report "War Over the Walrus" (air date September 1, 1992), accurately reflect what was said at this time.

7. See Marine Mammal Commission Annual Report for 2002, www.mmc .gov/species/pdf/ar2002pacificwalrus.pdf.

8. Alex deMarban, "Villagers Say Walrus Hunt Has Suffered Effects of Global Warming," Knight-Ridder/Tribune News Service, August 21, 2007.

9. See Rhett A. Butler, "Global Warming Could Doom the Walrus," mongabay.com, April 14, 2006, http://news.mongabay.com/2006/0413-walrus.html. See also Lee W. Cooper, et al., "Rapid Seasonal Sea-Ice Retreat in the Arctic Could Be Affecting Pacific Walrus (*Odobenus rosmarus divergens*) Recruitment," *Aquatic Mammals* 32, no. 1 (2006), pp. 98–102, and "News Release: Walrus Calves Stranded by

Melting Sea Ice," Woods Hole Oceanographic Institution, April 13, 2006, www.whoi.edu/page.do?pid=9779&tid=282&cid=12209&ct=162.

10. G. Carleton Ray, Jerry McCormick-Ray, Peter Berg, and Howard E. Epstein, "Pacific Walrus: Benthic Bioturbator of Beringia," *Journal of Experimental Marine Biology and Ecology* 330 (2006), pp. 403–419. See http://doc.nprb.org/web/BSIERP/Ray%20et%20al%202006%20walrus%20in%20the%20Bering%20Sea.pdf.

11. Robert Siegel, "Climate Changes Lives of Whalers in Alaska," *All Things Considered,* National Public Radio, September 17, 2007.

12. DeMarban, "Villagers Say Walrus Hunt Has Suffered Effects of Global Warming."

13. The Airborne Hunting Act prohibits shooting or attempting to shoot or harass any bird, fish, or other animal from an aircraft. Exceptions are allowed for protection of wildlife, livestock, and human life, and must be authorized via a state or federal permit or license.

Chapter Two: Walrus Forensic Investigation

1. From Paul L. Kirk, *Crime Investigation: Physical Evidence and the Police Laboratory* (New York: Interscience Publishers, 1953), p. 4, as quoted in "Criminalistics," American Academy of Forensic Sciences website at www.aafs.org/default.asp?section_id=resources&page_id=choosing_a_career#Criminalistics.

2. Some scientists now question the efficacy of this test, and others suggest it is effective only for fresh water and not salt water.

3. Memorandum from Ken Goddard, director, National Fish and Wildlife Forensics Laboratory, to Dave Purinton, assistant regional director–law enforcement, on "Walrus Investigation," June 4, 1990.

4. A walrus baculum might sell for US$50 in the immediate Arctic region and more than double that, US$125 or higher, farther afield.

5. Baculums are also found in other Alaskan species such as foxes, seals, and polar bears as well as in raccoons and minks.

6. Fibrin is an elastic, insoluble protein that forms a fibrous network over a wound that traps blood cells to help it clot.

7. This study was completed under Project Chariot. While not confirmed, information suggests it aimed to explore different scenarios for where one would look for a bomb if it got loose.

8. Edgar Espinoza, Bonnie Yates, Mary-Jacque Mann, et al., "Taphonomic Indicators Used to Infer Wasteful Subsistence Hunting in Northwest Alaska," *Anthropozoologica* no. 25–26 (1997), p. 111.

Chapter Three: Native Alaskan Solutions to Walrus Headhunting

1. Kenneth Goddard, Edgard Espinoza, and Richard Stroud, "Preliminary Investigations of Causes of Death and Stranding of Walrus (*Odobenus rosmarus*) in the Northern Bering Strait and Southern Chuckchi Sea," FWS, August 1990, pp. 9–10.

2. James W. Brooks, *North to Wolf Country: My Life Among the Creatures of Alaska* (Kenmore, Wash.: Epicenter Press, 2003), p. 214.

3. Craig Medred, "Ivory Sting Nabs 29," *Alaska Daily News,* February 13, 1992.

4. He was charged with six counts of illegally selling walrus ivory. He later pleaded guilty to two counts of illegally selling walrus ivory. His sentence included:

$1,000 fine, $100 special assessment, $2,577.50 restitution, and 12 months' imprisonment.

5. Sheila Toomey, "Expert Says Walrus Foul Witness Testifies Organs Are Too Contaminated to Eat," *Anchorage Daily News,* July 28, 1992, p. B1.

6. Sheila Toomey, "Wasted Walrus Meat Tainted, Defense Claims," *Anchorage Daily News,* July 22, 1992, p. A1.

7. Ibid.

8. Research to determine pollution levels and impact is ongoing. Fifteen years later, the EWC completed a review of available research. While more is known about toxins in whale and seal meat, less work has been done on walrus meat.

9. The Eskimo Walrus Commission is an organization of walrus-hunting communities, located from Barrow down to Bristol Bay, that advocates for continued use of the walrus and works with appropriate government agencies, including the U.S. Fish and Wildlife Service and Alaska Department of Fish and Game, to help perpetuate the species.

10. *United States of America, Plaintiff, vs. Glenn Iyahuk, Edgar Iyapana, Patrick Omiak, Dennis Soolook and Patrick Soolook, Defendants,* U.S. District Court, District of Alaska, Trial by Jury—7th Day, Transcript of Proceedings Before the Honorable Harry Branson, Case No. A92–033 CR, pp. 7–121.

11. Minutes, Eskimo Walrus Commission meeting, Anchorage, Alaska, October 13, 1992, p. 7.

12. Eskimo Walrus Commission Press Release, October 23, 1992.

13. Ibid.

14. Tim Woody, "Point Hope," *Alaska,* July 2003.

15. Diana Haecker, "Point Hope: Celebrating the Gift of Whales, Part III," *Canku Ota* (online newsletter celebrating Native America), August 9, 2003, Issue 93, see www.turtletrack.org/Issues03/Co08092003/CO_08092003_PointHopeWhaling-III.htm.

16. The lab found metal fragments in the neck of two sea lions, and a metal slug in the blubber of a third. These findings eliminated gunshot wounds, originally suspected to be the culprit, as the sea lions' cause of death.

17. David Hulen, "Outlaws Leave Walruses to Rot," *Anchorage Daily News,* June 16, 1996, p. A1.

18. Ibid.

19. David Hulen, "Walrus Hunters Protest," *Anchorage Daily News,* July 26, 1996, p. A1.

20. Letter from Brendan Kelly, research associate, University of Alaska–Fairbanks, to Mark Webb, July 30, 1996.

21. "Headless Walrus: A Few Changes Are in Order," *Anchorage Daily News,* August 6, 1996, p. B6.

22. Letter from Levi Cleveland, chairman, Robert Aqqaluk Newlin Sr. Memorial Trust, representing NANA Regional Elders Council (Northwest Arctic Borough), to David Allen, Regional Director, USFWS, Anchorage, September 10, 1996.

23. Ibid.

24. During the same time period in 1996, Special Agents Webb and C. J. Roberts also investigated walrus hunting in Kobuk. Because the village is more than 100 miles from the coast, there was a question about whether Kobuk residents were eligible to hunt walrus under the Marine Mammal Protection Act exemption because it applied to coastal-dwelling Native Alaskans. During the investigation, Webb and Roberts questioned a resident. Native Alaskan organizations later complained that Webb intimidated this resident. FWS disputed this charge. The agency noted the resident was cooperative, although his neighbors were abusive to the agents, and acknowledged that being questioned during a federal investiga-

tion can be imposing. It later discontinued the investigation because it determined that the Kobuk community had a history of subsistence harvest of marine mammals and that the Marine Mammal Protection Act exemption had no definition of coastal-dwelling communities.

25. Letter from Chuck Greene, mayor, Northwest Arctic Borough, to David Allen, regional director, USFWS, Anchorage, August 12, 1996.

26. Letter from Caleb Pungowiyi, director, Eskimo Walrus Commission, to David Allen, regional director, USFWS, Anchorage, December 9, 1996.

27. Ibid.

28. Letter from David Allen, regional director, USFWS, Anchorage, to Caleb Pungowiyi, director, Eskimo Walrus Commission, February 19, 1997.

29. Natalie Phillips, "Natives, Feds Work Out Way to Cool Heated Talk," *Anchorage Daily News,* October 19, 1996, p. D3.

30. Hulen, "Outlaws Leave Walruses to Rot."

31. Minutes, Eskimo Walrus Commission, Executive Committee Meeting, June 16, 2000, Nome, Alaska.

32. Eskimo Walrus Commission, *Pacific Walrus: Conserving Our Culture Through Traditional Management* (Nome: Kawerak, Inc., undated), p. 56.

33. Ibid., p. 64.

34. Ibid., p. 27.

35. Ibid., p. 20.

36. Ibid., p. 77.

37. Bill McKibben, *Wandering Home* (New York: Crown Publishers, 2005), pp. 115–16.

38. Author interview with Vera Metcalf, August 7, 2005.

39. Eskimo Walrus Commission, *Pacific Walrus,* p. 2.

40. Melissa Block, "Climate Changes Lives of Whalers in Alaska," *All Things Considered,* National Public Radio, September 20, 2007.

41. Eskimo Walrus Commission, *Pacific Walrus,* pp. 60–61.

42. Ibid., pp. 36 and 37.

43. Ibid., p. 37.

44. Minutes, Eskimo Walrus Commission Executive Committee Meeting, June 16, 2000, Nome, Alaska.

45. Minutes, Eskimo Walrus Commission Meeting, October 16–17, 1995, Anchorage; and Minutes, Eskimo Walrus Commission Executive Committee Meeting, March 12, 1996.

46. "Opinion: Walrus Ivory Headhunters Create Serious Concern," *Anchorage Daily News,* July 20, 1996, p. D8.

47. "Walrus Cases, May 2003," e-mail from Steve Oberholtzer to author, April 12, 2006.

48. Author interview with Steve Oberholtzer, April 12, 2006.

49. Nicole Tsong, "Gambell Walrus Hunter Receives Three-Year Sentence," *Anchorage Daily News,* January 6, 2005, p. B4.

50. "In January 2005, one hunter received 3 years in prison for felony possession violation and 12 months in prison for the MMPA violation, both running concurrently. The remaining 4 hunters collectively received 12 years probation, 800 hours community service and 120 days home confinement. They must also make presentation at 25 public hunter meetings and must salvage all parts of the walrus on their hunts." From "Walrus Cases," e-mail from Steve Oberholtzer to author, April 12, 2006.

51. Mary Pemberton, "Wasting Six Walruses Nets Barrow Man Seven Years," *Anchorage Daily News,* July 13, 2005, p. B9.

52. While residents from two Inupiat villages in Norton Sound agreed that they had

never seen so many, others argued that the high number of headless carcasses might not be greater than in previous years but instead be the result of more reporting because they were washing ashore closer to communities.

53. Alex De Marban, "Headless Walruses Littering Northwest Alaska Beaches," *Anchorage Daily News,* August 15, 2007.

54. High-altitude (20,000 feet) thermal infrared scanning allowed teams to count walrus accurately based on their thermal signature (with, say, ten walrus always registering a specific magnitude) as well as capture an area five times larger than previous surveys. They also could now account for walrus in the water at any one time because, using wet-dry satellite sensor tags, they had developed a record of how much time walrus spent in and out of the water.

55. Similar to polar bears, these dual risks prompted a 2008 petition (and lawsuit for failure to process it) by the Center for Biological Diversity to protect Pacific walrus under the Endangered Species Act. In May 2008, the polar bear was listed as threatened, the first time the act protected a species due to climate change. While a decision on walrus is still years down the road, success would limit oil development and not subsistence hunting.

56. Eskimo Walrus Commission, *Pacific Walrus,* p. 23.

57. Haecker, "Point Hope: Celebrating the Gift of Whales, Part III."

58. Robert Siegel, "Climate Changes Lives of Whalers in Alaska," *All Things Considered,* National Public Radio, September 17, 2007.

59. Author interview with Al Crane, August 2005, and reiterated June 19, 2008.

Chapter Four: Busted for Bear Galls

1. Most vertebrates have gallbladders, although some, like horses, whales, elephants, and some birds, do not. However, one can always obtain bile from the biliary duct leading from the liver to the intestine. Only vertebrates have a large requirement for cholesterol to serve as a nerve insulator (to allow conduction of nerve impulses over a longer distance). Most invertebrates cannot synthesize cholesterol and do not utilize enough of it to need a specialized system to dispose of it.

2. "Bear Trade Galls Conservationists," *TRAFFIC Newsletter* 11, no. 1 (April 1991).

3. Bear bile has been chemically synthesized from cow bile since 1955, with about 200 metric tons consumed annually and about 10 tons in North America.

4. Tim Phillips and Philip Wilson, *The Bear Bile Business: The Global Trade in Bear Products from China to Asia and Beyond* (London: World Society for the Protection of Animals, October 2002), p. 16.

5. Kalinga Seneviratne, "Traditional Medicine Often Lauded but Neglected," Third World Network, December 8, 2000, www.twnside.org.sg/title/lauded.htm.

6. Richard Ellis, *Tiger Bone & Rhino Horn: The Destruction of Wildlife for Traditional Chinese Medicine* (Washington, D.C.: Island Press/Shearwater Books, 2005), p. 35.

7. Ibid., pp. 39–40.

8. Qian Jia, *Traditional Chinese Medicine Could Make "Health for One" True,* Institute of Scientific and Technical Information (China), study commissioned for World Health Organization, Commission on Intellectual Property Rights, Innovation and Public Health, Geneva, 2005, p. 49. See www.who.int/intellectualproperty/studies/Jia.pdf.

9. Ellis, *Tiger Bone & Rhino Horn,* p. 38.

10. Author interview with Jill Robinson, July 17, 2007.

11. Phillips and Wilson, *The Bear Bile Business,* p. 28.
12. The U.S. Fish and Wildlife Service Forensics Lab has shown that the concentration of bile acids is different for farmed bears versus wild ones.
13. Robin Meadows, "Smuggling Bear Galls," *Chem Matters,* December 1994, p. 6.
14. Douglas F. Williamson, *In the Black: Status, Management, and Trade of the American Black Bear (Ursus americanus) in North America* (Washington, D.C.: World Wildlife Fund and TRAFFIC USA, 2002), p. 14.
15. Ibid., pp. 2 and 12.
16. Sport-hunting of black bears is allowed in twenty-seven of the forty-one U.S. states with bears and all eleven of the Canadian provinces and territories with bears.
17. Williamson, *In the Black,* pp. 41–42.
18. A gallbladder's size is not determined by the age and size of the bear. Bear cubs can have large ones and large bears can have small ones. Consequently, cubs are often targeted for the trade.
19. Williamson, *In the Black,* p. 48.
20. Ibid.
21. "Senses of the Black Bear," www.americanbear.org/senses.htm.
22. Gary Brown, *The Great Bear Almanac* (New York: Lyons Press, 1993). Referenced by "Senses of the Black Bear," www.americanbear.org/senses.htm.
23. "Senses of the Black Bear," www.americanbear.org/senses.htm. The Jacobson's organ, also called vomeronasal organ (in other mammals) and vomeronasal pit (in snakes), is used to detect trace quantities of chemicals. Snakes and other reptiles flick substances onto the organ with their tongues while some mammals (e.g., cats) curl their upper lip (as in a sneer), called the Flehmen reaction, to expose the organs for chemical sensing. In mammals, it is also used for communication within the same species through the emission and reception of chemical signals called pheromones. While humans don't display the Flehmen reaction, recent studies have demonstrated that Jacobson's organ functions in other mammals to detect pheromones and to sample low concentrations of certain nonhuman chemicals in the air. There are indications that Jacobson's organ may be stimulated in pregnant women, perhaps partially accounting for an improved sense of smell during pregnancy and possibly implicated in morning sickness. See "Jacobson's Organ and the Sixth Sense," in *Your Guide to Chemistry* by Anne Marie Helmenstine, Ph.D., in http://chemistry.about.com/cs/medical/a/aa051601a.htm.
24. Peter Tyson, "Secrets of Hibernation," NOVA Online, www.pbs.org/wgbh/nova/satoyama/hibernation2.html.
25. Profile of Ethnic Origin and Visible Minorities for Census, Metropolitan Areas and Census Agglomerations, 2006 Census, from Wikipedia, "Demographics of Vancouver," retrieved from https://enwikipedia.org/wiki/Demographics_of_Vancouver.
26. Brown, *The Great Bear Almanac,* p. 255. Major consuming countries of bear gallbladders include South Korea, China, Hong Kong, Japan, Singapore, and Taiwan.
27. *Traditional Medicine,* World Health Organization, Fact sheet No. 134, Revised May 2003, www.who.int/mediacentre/factsheets/fs134/en/print.html.
28. Ibid.
29. *Traditional Chinese Medicine Could Make "Health for One" True,* p. 20.
30. Teresa Castle, "State Battles Lucrative Bear Bile Trade," *San Francisco Chronicle,* April 25, 2005, see www.sfgate.com.
31. Judy Mills and Christopher Servheen, *The Asian Trade in Bears and Bear Parts* (Washington, D.C.: World Wildlife Fund and TRAFFIC USA, 1991), pp. 87 and 91.
32. Merilyn P. Twiss and Vernon G. Thomas, "Illegal Harvests of Black Bears, Sale of

Black Bear Parts, and the Canadian Legislative Response," *Wildlife Society Bulletin* 27, no. 3 (Autumn 1999), pp. 692–97.

33. Mills and Servheen, *The Asian Trade in Bears and Bear Parts,* pp. 87 and 91.

34. Port of Vancouver, *Port Plan Update,* May 2003, p. 7, www.portvancouver.com/the_port/docs/LOWRES%20Growth%20Opportunities.pdf.

35. Human-wildlife conflicts like this one happen the world over as people move into wild areas and encroach on what used to be the animals' sole territory. Sharing the space often results in tension, like wolves marauding ranchers' cattle in the American west, elephants raiding farmers' crops in southern Africa, or bears prowling city trash heaps in Vancouver. The last-resort solution, killing the problem animal, is an unpleasant but often necessary task.

36. Prices vary widely. Hunters tend to receive the lowest amounts, with middlemen and retailers each receiving increasingly more. According to "Appendix 15: Reported Prices of Black Bears and Black Bear Parts in the United States, 1992 and 1996 Surveys," in Williamson, *In the Black,* p. 152, hunters received $20 to $300 for gallbladders, while middlemen and retailers each received more. Also, in general, the farther away from the source, the more money charged. Hence, prices in South Korea are astronomical.

Chapter Five: Bear Bile . . . or Not?

1. Judy A. Mills and Christopher Servheen, *The Asian Trade in Bears and Bear Parts,* (Washington, D.C.: World Wildlife Fund and TRAFFIC USA, 1991), p. 84.

2. Keith Highley, *The American Bear Parts Trade: A State-by-State Analysis* (Washington, D.C.: The Humane Society of the United States, April 1996), p. 11.

3. The operation was called Operation SOUP by the National Park Service. FWS referred to the same operation as Operation Ursus.

4. Highley, *The American Bear Parts Trade,* p. 9.

5. Ibid.

6. Ibid., pp. 9–10.

7. Tim Phillips and Philip Wilson, *The Bear Bile Business: The Global Trade in Bear Products from China to Asia and Beyond* (London: World Society for the Protection of Animals, 2002), p. 77.

8. A. C. MacDonald and C. N. Williams, "Studies of Bile Lipids and Bile Acids of Wild North American Black Bears in Nova Scotia, Showing a High Content of Ursodeoxycholic Acid," *Journal of Surgical Research* 38 (1985), p. 173.

9. Ibid.

10. Subsequently, the use of UDC as a human medicine has become a multimillion-dollar industry.

11. MacDonald and Williams, "Studies of Bile Lipids," p. 173.

12. Ibid., p. 177.

13. Author interview with Lee Hagey, February 27, 2007.

14. Author written communication with Lee Hagey, July 31, 2007.

15. Criminalistics Examination Report, Lab Case # 90–0144, Agency Case #2701 AL, USFWS, Division of Law Enforcement, National Fish and Wildlife Forensics Laboratory, September 24, 1990.

16. Author interview with Ken Goddard, April 18, 2003.

17. Percentage calculated from data contained in FWS annual reports.

Chapter Six: The Impact of Bear Investigation

1. Regulatory Intelligence Data, "Company President Pleads Guilty to Caviar Smuggling Conspiracy," May 21, 2004.
2. "Caviar Company President Pleads Guilty," *Federal Wildlife Officer* 15, no. 3 (Fall 2002).
3. FWS Press Release, "Caviar Smuggler Pleads Guilty: Wildlife Inspectors Found 1,700 Pounds in Mislabeled Containers," U.S. Fish and Wildlife Service, March 30, 2001.
4. Letter from Jim Wolfe, Scientific Crime Detection Laboratory, Department of Public Safety, State of Alaska, Anchorage, Alaska, to Wayne Ferguson, chief serologist, USFWS Forensics Lab, Ashland, Oregon, dated January 7, 1991.
5. This and the following quotations are taken from the court transcript of the proceedings: "*Regina v. Sang Ho Kim,* Proceedings at Trial," in the Provincial Court of British Columbia, before the Honourable Judge W. G. MacDonald, Surrey B.C., April 26, 1994, File No. 60597C.
6. The counts against Kim were: 6 counts of unlawful possession of dead wildlife (Wildlife Act section 33 bracket 2); 2 counts of failed to complete return on wildlife (Wildlife Act section 71 bracket 2)—meaning he didn't submit his reports; 1 count of failure to keep record of wildlife received (Wildlife Act section 71 bracket 1 bracket e)—meaning he didn't keep complete records of what he purchased from others; 2 counts of fur trade without a license (section 72 bracket 1); and 1 count of failure to obtain fur trader license for business (section 72 bracket 3). One of the charges of failed to complete return on wildlife was dismissed.
7. Christopher Servheen, "Comments on the Trade in Bears and Bear Parts," October 22, 1995. Written submission included as part of evidence for Kim case.
8. Andy Ivens, "Sale of Bear Parts Nets $10,400 Fine," *Vancouver Province,* January 15, 1996, p. A6.
9. "Slap on the Paw," editorial, *Vancouver Province,* January 15, 1996, p. A14.
10. Also discussed but rejected at this meeting was a proposal to uplist Eurasian brown bears (*Ursus arctos*) from Appendix II to Appendix I (Prop. 10.24).
11. CITES Res. Conf. 10.8.
12. Senator Mitch McConnell, Statement before the Senate Environment and Public Works Committee, on S. 263, the Bear Protection Act, July 7, 1998.
13. Ray Schoenke, Testimony before the Subcommittee on Fisheries, Wildlife and Oceans of the House Committee on Natural Resources on HR 5534, The Bear Protection Act of 2008, March 11, 2008.
14. Debates about whether legal trade increases or reduces the illegal trade are heated and ongoing with respect to numerous species, such as elephants. Many stakeholders argue that legal trade helps to convert illegal trade and better control it (similar to arguments regarding legalization of marijuana), and provides room for socioeconomic incentives that encourage voluntary conservation and are much more effective than traditional command-and-control methods (such as bans) of regulating trade.
15. Jill Robinson, "Bear Farming Across Asia: An Animal Welfare Perspective," from *Proceedings of the Third International Symposium on Trade in Bear Parts,* D. Williamson and M. J. Phipps, eds. (Washington, D.C.: TRAFFIC East Asia, Ministry of Environment of Republic of Korea, and IUCN/SSC Bear Specialist Group, 2001), p. 110.
16. Judy A. Mills and Christopher Servheen, *The Asian Trade in Bears and Bear Parts,* (Washington, D.C.: World Wildlife Fund and TRAFFIC USA, 1991), p. 15.
17. Author interview with Jill Robinson, July 17, 2007. Also described by Patricia L.

Howard, "A New Phase for China's Moon Bears," IMPACT Press, February-March 2003, at www.impactpress.com/articles/febmar03/moonbears2303 .html.

18. "Interview with Jill Robinson, Founder and CEO of Animals Asia Foundation," Mad About Shanghai, June 19, 2007, at www.madaboutshanghai.com/2007/06/interview_with_.html.

19. Judy Mills, "Milking the Bear Trade," *International Wildlife,* May/June 1992, p. 44.

20. Janet Raloff, "A Galling Business: The Inhumane Exploitation of Bears for Traditional Asian Medicine," *Science News Online* 168, no. 16 (week of October 15, 2005).

21. See www.wspa-international.org/inside.asp?cnewsID=84&campaignType=3.

22. Speech by Wang Wei, deputy director of Department of Wildlife Conservation, under the State Forestry Administration, January 12, 2006. See http://au.china-embassy.org/eng/sgfyrth/t236846.htm or www.china.org.cn/e-news/news 060112–1.htm.

23. Mills, "Milking the Bear Trade," p. 44.

24. Raloff, "A Galling Business."

25. Speech by Wang Wei, January 12, 2006.

26. See www.animalsasia.org/index.php?module=2&menupos=7&submenupos= 3&lg=en.

27. Scarlett Oi Lan Pong, Dr. Yan Wo Lo, and Dr. Ka Cheong Ho, "Herbal Alternatives to Bear Bile," in *Proceedings of the Third International Symposium on Trade in Bear Parts,* pp. 156–57.

28. Grace Ge Gabriel, "A Bitter Medicine: The Use of Bear Bile in China," *Proceedings of the Third International Symposium on Trade in Bear Parts,* p. 120.

29. "Support from the TM Community," Heal without Harm, Animals Asia website, www.animnalsasia.org/index.php?modul=6&menupos-4&submenupos=&lg=en.

30. Author interview with Ed Espinoza, June 5, 2007.

31. "Roundtable Discussion," *Proceedings of the Third International Symposium on Trade in Bear Parts,* p. 165.

32. Mills and Servheen, *The Asian Trade in Bears and Bear Parts,* pp. 94–95.

33. Zhao Huanxin, "Extraction of Bear Bile 'Painless, Necessary,'" *China Daily,* January 13, 2006. See www.chinadaily.com.cn/english/doc/2006–01/13/content_511872.htm.

34. In 1993, China banned all trade in tiger bone and rhino horn.

35. Jill Robinson, "Cruelty Doesn't Cure: Working to Replace the Use of Animals in Traditional Oriental Medicine," unpublished paper.

36. Report on Implementing Resolution Conf.12.5 of CITES, prepared by CITES Management Authority, People's Republic of China, CoP14 Doc. 52 Annex 1, see www.cites.org/common/cop/14/doc/E14–52A01.pdf.

37. CoP14, Decision 14.69, see www.cites.org/eng/dec/valid14/14_65–72.shtml.

38. Mills, "Milking the Bear Trade," p. 42.

39. Jane Macartney, "Siphoning Bear Bile for Medicine Is Painless, says China," *The Times* of London, January 13, 2006.

40. Mills, "Milking the Bear Trade," p. 44.

41. Lila Buckley, "Conference on Traditional Chinese Medicine Marks Shift Towards Global Market, Raises Concerns About Social and Ecological Impact," Worldwatch Institute, www.worldwatch.org, October 12, 2005, see www.worldwatch .org/node/47/print.

42. Jia Hepeng, "Traditional Medicine 'Threatens China's Biodiversity,'" Science and Development Network, December 20, 2004, see: www.scidev.net/en/news/traditional-medicine-threatens-chinas-biodiversi.html.

43. "Traditional Chinese Medicine Exports Up 10.27% Last Year," Gov.cn (Chinese

Governments Official Web Portal), February 10, 2006, see ww.gov.cn/english /2006–02/10/content_185110.htm.

44. "Traditional Medicine Designated Strategic Sector," *Asia Times Online,* www.atimes.com/atimes/China_Business/GK15Cb03.html.

45. Malia Politzer, "Eastern Medicine Goes West," Opinion, *Wall Street Journal,* September 14, 2007.

46. Margot Higgins, "China Pledges Sustainable Trade in Traditional Medicine," Environment News Network, November 4, 1999.

47. Hepeng, "Traditional Medicine 'Threatens China's Biodiversity.'"

48. Buckley, "Conference on Traditional Chinese Medicine."

49. Ibid.

50. "Promoting Sustainable Traditional Chinese Medicine," News and Publications, World Wildlife Fund, April 26, 2006, www.panda.org/about_wwf/ where _we_work/asia_pacific/where/china/news/index.cf.

51. Buckley, "Conference on Traditional Chinese Medicine."

52. Higgins, "China Pledges Sustainable Trade in Traditional Medicine."

Chapter Seven: The Feather Artifacts

1. There are numerous correct spellings for Indian tribes (such as Rikbaktsa for Rikbatsa), with many of the names meaning "the human beings."

2. "Rikbatsa," see www.socioambiental.org/pib/epienglish/rikbatsa/rikbatsa .shtm.

3. Ibid.

4. University of Michigan, Department of Zoology, "*Ara macao:* Scarlet Macaw," Animal Diversity Web, http://animaldiversity.ummz.umich.edu/site/accounts/information/Ara_macao.html.

5. "Indigenous People in Brazil," see www.socioambiental.org/pib/english/whwh how/index.shtm.

6. Instituto Socioambiental, "General Table of the Indigenous People in Brazil," Indigenous Peoples in Brazil, see www.socioambiental.org/pib/english/whwh how/table.asp.

7. For a detailed description of this ceremony, see Barbara Braun, *Arts of the Amazon* (London: Thames and Hudson, 1995), pp. 98–102.

8. Figures are from USFWS, Office of Law Enforcement, Annual Report FY2007, September 2008, p. 32, see www.fws.gov/le/pdffiles/AnnualReportFY2007. pdf.

9. Where no wildlife inspectors are posted, suspect packages are identified by officers from the border services, previously the U.S. Customs Service and now the Department of Homeland Security.

10. The Amazon rain forest is located in nine countries: Brazil (60 percent), Bolivia (230,000 square miles), Ecuador (11 million ha = 42,000 square miles), Peru (69 million ha = 266,000 square miles), Colombia, Venezuela, Suriname, French Guiana, and Guyana.

11. *1st National Report on the Traffic of Wild Animals* (Brazil: RENCTAS, 2001), pp. 31–33.

12. Anthony Faiola, "Smuggling's Wild Side in Brazil: Animal Trafficking Sucks the Life from Amazon Rain Forest," *Washington Post,* December 9, 2001.

13. Braun, *Arts of the Amazon,* p. 15.

14. Alan Riding, "France's New Look at Brazil's Indians," *New York Times,* April 26, 2005. See www.nytimes.com/2005/04/26/arts/design/26indi.html?_r=1&page wanted=print&position=&oref=slogin.

15. *1st National Report on the Traffic of Wild Animals,* pp. 6 and 37.

16. Francesca Colombo, "Environment: Animal Trafficking—A Cruel Billion-Dollar Business," Inter Press Service English News Wire, September 6, 2003, see http://ipsnews.net/africa/interna.asp?idnews=20005.

17. Howard Youth, "The Plight of Birds," WorldWatch, May/June 2002.

18. Christine Eckstrom, "Homeless Macaws?" International Wildlife, September 1, 1994.

19. This and subsequent messages come directly from copies of the e-mails as contained in the case files for this investigation, INV #501000029 (Macaw Feathers).

20. Braun, Arts of the Amazon, pp. 51, 58, and 59.

21. Portaria no 93 of 7 July 1998. The law also requires anyone who transports an item that contains wildlife parts from species listed under CITES Appendix II to have a CITES permit issued by IBAMA.

22. IBAMA fax to FWS Office of Law Enforcement, January 17, 2001.

23. To set up the mail covers, LeClair first had to identify the relevant addresses. With local agents surveying the post office, he discovered four boxes at one Gainesville, Florida, post office and another at a downtown post office in the name of a friend.

Chapter Eight: Fly-by-Night Evidence

1. The genus (plural form, genera) is the second-lowest category in the taxonomic hierarchy, which organizes relationships between organisms. The highest level, kingdom (e.g., plant or animal), is very general while the lower levels are increasingly specific. Categories from highest to lowest are: kingdom; phylum (e.g., vertebrates); class (e.g., birds); order (e.g., songbirds); family (e.g., thrushes); genus; and species. A genus may contain several species, and a family, several genera.

2. Author interview with Pepper Trail, October 10, 2007.

3. The lab's standard collection is constantly growing. As of the end of 2008, it included 8,000 specimens and over 1,100 species in the bird collection.

4. While not asked in this case, the lab often establishes the number of individual animals contained in an article. It does this by counting the number of repeated elements, like upper-right canine teeth or outermost primary wing feather, for which an animal only has one. From this, the lab determines the minimum number of individuals, or MNI.

5. John Kricher, A Neotropical Companion: An Introduction to the Animals, Plants and Ecosystems of the New World Tropics (Princeton, N.J.: Princeton University Press, 1997), p. 312.

Chapter Nine: Buyer Beware

1. Author interview with Dan LeClair, June 9, 2006.

2. Once the U.S. marshals transfer a prisoner to the Bureau of Prisons, the prisoners are sent to facilities based on openings. Hrabovsky could have been sent to any federal prison facility in the country that wasn't a maximum security facility. In Hrabovsky's case, he was sent to South Carolina.

3. Jacqueline Trescott, "U.S. Charges Smithsonian Secretary; Small's Art Collection Contains Illegal Feathers," Washington Post, January 21, 2004, p. A1.

4. James Bone, "Heard the One About the Anthropologist Sent to the Amazon as a Punishment?" The Times, June 17, 2005.

5. Jacqueline Trescott, "The Feathers That Caused a Flap; Case Against Smithsonian Secretary Was Three Years in the Making," Washington Post, January 22, 2004, p. C1.

6. Michael Kilian, "Smithsonian Chief Guilty in Rare Bird Case: Plea Bargain over Illegal Feathers Gets Small Probation," *Chicago Tribune,* January 24, 2004, p. 10.
7. Bone, "Heard the One About the Anthropologist?"
8. Small offered to spend his one hundred hours of community service working on reauthorization of the Endangered Species Act (ESA), a key piece of legislation to prevent illegal wildlife trade, but the prosecution fought that proposal, saying that it undermined the ESA to allow the defendant to work to change the law that he violated.
9. Author interview with FWS Special Agent Allen Hundley, August 7, 2008.
10. The $1 million figure comes from author interview with Matthew Bryant, August 8, 2008. Prosecutor quote is from Rudolph Bush, "2 Charged in Smuggling Case—Gallery Owners Had Art Made of Protected Animals, Officials Say," *Chicago Tribune,* January 11, 2006.
11. Author interview with Matthew Bryant, August 8, 2008.
12. Ibid.
13. Associated Press, "Government Working to Get Artifacts for Museum," *Naples Daily News,* July 3, 2003.
14. IBAMA fax, January 17, 2001.
15. *Pindorama* means "land of the palms" and is what Brazil's Indians used to call the country before the Portuguese arrived.
16. Author interview with Jorge Pontes, August 7, 2008.
17. Author interview with Jorge Pontes, August 1, 2008.
18. "Wildlife Smuggling Rises in Brazil," BBC News, November 13, 2001. See http://news.bbc.co.uk/1/hi/world/americas/1653034.stm.
19. Scott Wallace, "Last of the Amazon," *National Geographic,* January 2007.
20. Author interview with Jorge Pontes, August 1, 2008.
21. Anthony Faiola, "Smuggling's Wild Side in Brazil: Animal Trafficking Sucks the Life from Amazon Rain Forest," *Washington Post,* December 9, 2001.
22. While not asked to do so for this investigation, the lab can determine the minimum number of individuals (MNI) involved. For instance, the lab could have used the canine teeth in the Bororo shaman's necklace to estimate the number of jaguars killed for that article because there is only one canine for each position (top right, bottom right, top left, bottom left). In this case, Sims would have said the MNI is one, meaning she had one complete set of teeth, and could only say one animal was involved. For birds, a similar calculation can be made by using feathers that have unique characteristics for particular positions, like eagle wing feathers.
23. Andrew Hay, "Brazil Trains Environmental Police to Guard Amazon," Reuters, November 17, 2004. See http://rainforests.mongabay.com/amazon/external_nov04.html.
24. Wallace, "Last of the Amazon."
25. Hay, "Brazil Trains Environmental Police to Guard Amazon."
26. Associated Press, "U.S. Wildlife Experts to Teach Brazilian Environmental Police," February 14, 2005, www.enn.com/top_stories/article/966/print.

Chapter Ten: Conclusion

1. Quote from Stephen Colbert, *The Colbert Report,* October, 18, 2007.
2. General Accounting Office, "Wildlife Protection: Fish and Wildlife Service's Inspection Program Needs Strengthening," GAO/RCED-95-8, Washington, D.C., December 1994, p. 33. Data from U.S. Fish and Wildlife Service, Office of Law Enforcement, Annual Report FY 2007, September 2008, p. 33, shows that pun-

ishments for all of FWS's investigations averaged just $1,600 in fines or civil penalties and less than one-day prison sentences for each case. The number of investigative cases worked by FWS special agents and wildlife inspectors during FY 2007 totaled 12,177 and generated $14.2 million in fines, $5.3 million in civil penalties, 31 years in prison, and 536 years of probation.

3. According to the March 5, 2008, written testimony of William Clark to the U.S. House of Representatives Committee on Natural Resources, the August 2006 smuggling of 2,409 kilograms (5,300 pounds) of raw ivory and 17,928 hanko signature seals made from ivory (385 kilograms, or 847 pounds), together worth 1 billion yen ($9.4 million) resulted in a suspended sentence and an 800,000-yen ($7,500) fine for the perpetrator. Similarly, the April 2000 attempt to smuggle 492 kilograms (over 1,080 pounds) of illegal elephant ivory into Osaka, Japan, resulted in a 300,000-yen ($2,700) fine—less than 2 percent of the shipment's wholesale value—for one of the two people convicted and a suspended sentence for the other.

4. Wildlife Alliance, "Bangkok Luxury Store Owner Convicted for Wildlife Trafficking," Environmental News Network, August 28, 2007, www.enn.com /wildlife/article/22405.

5. Indonesian Government, untitled (Asian Big Cats: Indonesia Country Report), CITES SC 57 Doc. 31.1 Annex 5, July 2008, p. 12.

6. The federal wildlife law enforcement budget for FY 2007 was $57.3 million. It last received a significant increase in FY 2001, when the budget went from $39 million the previous year to almost $50 million.

7. CITES, "Interpretation and Implementation of the Convention, Compliance and Enforcement Issues: Enforcement Matters," CoP14 Doc. 25, presented to CITES 14th Conference of Parties, Hague, Netherlands, June 3–15, 2007, p. 5.

8. CITES, "National Wildlife Trade Policy Reviews," SC57 Doc. 17, presented to 57th Standing Committee Meeting, Geneva, July 14–18, 2008.

9. Federal Bureau of Investigation, "The FBI Work Force: By the Numbers," August 25, 2004, see www.fbi.gov/page2/aug04/workforce082504.htm.

10. Drug Enforcement Administration, "DEA Staffing and Budget," see www.usdoj.gov/dea/agency/staffing.htm.

11. Federal Bureau of Investigation, "Law Enforcement Personnel," from Crime in the United States: 2004, U.S. Department of Justice, Table 74, see www.fbi .gov/ucr/cius_04/law_enforcement_personnel/index.html.

12. New York and Newark operate together as one "designated" port with two locations.

13. U.S. Customs and Border Patrol, "This Is CBP," see www.cbp.gov/xp/cgov/ about/mission/cbp_is.xml.

14. Figures are for fiscal year 2007. See U.S. Fish and Wildlife Service, Office of Law Enforcement, Annual Report FY 2007, September 2008, p. 32.

15. Author interview with Terry Grosz, August 9, 2004. According to the U.S. Fish and Wildlife Service, Office of Law Enforcement, Annual Report FY 2007, September 2008, in FY 2007 the designated port of New York (the busiest port of entry for wildlife trade) received 32,000 declared wildlife shipments and Los Angeles (the second busiest) received 24,400 declared wildlife shipments. Of these, about 18 percent were physically inspected.

16. Sandra Cleva, "Enforcement Starts with Wildlife Inspectors," Endangered Species Update, January 1, 2006.

17. Michael D. Lemonick, "Environment: Animal Genocide, Mob Style: A New Report Says Organized Crime Is Muscling In on the Illegal Wildlife Trade," Time, November 14, 1994.

18. Hugh Muir, "Yard Plan to Halve Size of Wildlife Crime Unit Angers Campaigners," *The Guardian,* May 24, 2007. See www.guardian.co.uk/uk/2007/may/24/animalwelfare.ukcrime.
19. Anthony Faiola, "Smuggling's Wild Side in Brazil: Animal Trafficking Sucks the Life from Amazon Rain Forest," *Washington Post,* December 9, 2001.
20. Ibid.
21. Author interview with Terry Grosz, August 9, 2004.
22. Samuel Wasser, William Clark, Ofir Drori, et al., "Combating the Illegal Trade in African Elephant Ivory with DNA Forensics," *Conservation Biology* 22, no. 4, 1065–71. Also reported in the March 2007 *Proceedings of the National Academy of Sciences.*
23. Australian scientists have developed a DNA test for bear bile to be used by agents in the field for detection of illicit bear bile and gallbladders. In the United States, field testing is not encouraged. For instance, police may conduct a field sobriety test but the Breathalyzer results are then sent to a forensic lab for analysis. Case precedents suggest that results from field tests would not be admitted as evidence in a U.S. court of law.
24. U.S. Fish and Wildlife Service, "Wildlife Forensics Acknowledged as Unique Field," *Fish and Wildlife News,* November/December 1999, p. 10.

INDEX

Page numbers in *italics* refer to illustrations.